Disinfection and Decontamination

A Practical Handbook

Disinfection and Decontamination

A Practical Handbook

Edited by
Jeanne Moldenhauer

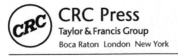

CRC Press
Taylor & Francis Group
Boca Raton London New York

CRC Press is an imprint of the
Taylor & Francis Group, an **informa** business

CRC Press
Taylor & Francis Group
6000 Broken Sound Parkway NW, Suite 300
Boca Raton, FL 33487-2742

First issued in paperback 2023

© 2019 by Taylor & Francis Group, LLC
CRC Press is an imprint of Taylor & Francis Group, an Informa business

No claim to original U.S. Government works

ISBN-13: 978-0-8153-7901-0 (hbk)
ISBN-13: 978-1-03-265315-0 (pbk)
ISBN-13: 978-1-351-21702-6 (ebk)

DOI: 10.1201/9781351217026

Library of Congress Cataloging-in-Publication Data

Names: Moldenhauer, Jeanne, editor.
Title: Disinfection and decontamination : a practical handbook / editor,
Jeanne Moldenhauer.
Other titles: Disinfection and decontamination (Moldenhauer)
Description: Boca Raton : Taylor & Francis, [2019] | Includes bibliographical
references and index. |
Identifiers: LCCN 2018031124 (print) | LCCN 2018031933 (ebook) | ISBN
9781351217019 (Adobe PDF) | ISBN 9781351217002 (ePub) | ISBN 9781351216999
(Mobipocket) | ISBN 9780815379010 (hardback : alk. paper) | ISBN
9781351217026 (ebook)
Subjects: | MESH: Disinfection--methods | Decontamination--methods |
Anti-Infective Agents--therapeutic use | Infection Control--methods |
Biofilms
Classification: LCC RA761 (ebook) | LCC RA761 (print) | NLM WA 240 | DDC
614.4/8--dc23
LC record available at https://lccn.loc.gov/2018031124

Visit the Taylor & Francis Web site at
http://www.taylorandfrancis.com

and the CRC Press Web site at
http://www.crcpress.com

Contents

Editor

Jeanne Moldenhauer, Vice-President of Excellent Pharma Consulting, has more than 30 years' experience in the pharmaceutical industry. She chaired the Environmental Monitoring/Microbiology Interest Group of the Parenteral Drug Association (PDA) for more than 15 years, served on the Scientific Advisory Board of PDA for 20 years, founded the Rapid Microbiology User's Group™, and is a member of the American Society for Quality and the Regulatory Affairs Professionals Society. She is the author/editor of many books, including *Steam Sterilization: A Practitioner's Guide, Laboratory Validation: A Practitioner's Guide, Environmental Monitoring: A Comprehensive Handbook Volumes 1–8, Contamination Control Volumes 1–5* (with Russ Madsen), *Systems-Based Inspections for Pharmaceutical Manufacturers, Preparing for an FDA Inspection: Review of Warning Letters (Sterile and Non-Sterile), Biological Indicators*, and numerous book chapters and magazine articles.

Contributors

Christine Chan
Accuratus Lab Services
Eagan, Minnesota

Brian G. Hubka
Contamination Prevention Technologies, Inc.
Las Vegas, Nevada

Beth Kroeger
Steris Corporation
St. Louis, Missouri

Joe McCall, SM (NRCM)
Steris Corporation
St. Louis, Missouri

Jeanne Moldenhauer
Excellent Pharma Consulting, Inc.
Mundelein, Illinois

Jim Polarine, MA
Steris Corporation
St. Louis, Missouri

Dave Rottjakob
Accuratus Lab Services
Eagan, Minnesota

Tim Sandle
Pharmaceutical Microbiologist
St Albans, United Kingdom

Art Vellutato, Jr.
Veltek Associates, Inc.
Malvern, Pennsylvania

1 Introduction

Jeanne Moldenhauer

CONTENTS

1.1 BACKGROUND

Most regulated industries have experienced problems with contamination. Contamination comes in many forms, e.g., microbial, viral, endotoxin, chemical, or particulate. This book is focused on many topics that describe types of microbial and viral contamination and how they may be addressed using disinfection procedures, sanitization procedures, sterilization procedures, and a variety of new technologies. There are even some technologies that can prevent contamination from specific types of organisms for specified periods of time.

While the types and levels of contamination may be different in foods, devices, drugs, and biologics, many of the ways to deal with the contamination are the same. Many of the issues in using these disinfection and decontamination processes are the same for each different type of product.

This book describes a variety of different ways to perform disinfection, how to qualify disinfectants and preservatives, new technologies for decontamination or sterilization, and sterilization methods. All of the chapters will provide guidance for the development of your contamination control program at your facility.

1.2 REGULATORY ISSUES WITH DISINFECTION AND DECONTAMINATION

In recent years, there have been many significant issues with contamination across the regulated industries. Some of the predominant cases are described below.

1.2.1 THE NEW ENGLAND COMPOUNDING CENTER (NECC)

There was a major meningitis outbreak that was attributed to the New England Compounding Center (NECC) in Massachusetts in 2012. There were reports of over 800 individuals sickened with meningitis and 76 deaths. This outbreak of meningitis affected multiple states and it was investigated by the Centers for Disease Control (CDC), the Food and Drug Administration (FDA), and the state and local health departments. As a result, it was determined that the outbreak was linked to a contaminated steroid injection produced by NECC. This product was manufactured by NECC, which is designated as a compounding pharmacy. This company is only authorized to create specific formulations of drugs to meet the needs of individual patients and in response to individual prescriptions (Moldenhauer, 2017).

As a result of this outbreak, many different laws and requirements changed. Additionally, legal actions were taken against employees of NECC (Moldenhauer, 2017).

1.2.2 FOOD RECALLS

There were numerous food recalls, and a few of them are listed here.

1.2.2.1 Fieldbrook Foods Corporation Announces a Voluntary Recall of Orange Cream Bars for Possible Health Risk (2018)

Fieldbrook Foods Corporation of Dunkirk, New York, issued a voluntary recall of 20 cases of the Tops brand of Orange Cream Bars and 320 cases of the Meijer Purple

Cow brand Orange Cream Bars due to the possibility that the product may be contaminated with *Listeria monocytogenes*. Consumption of food contaminated with *Listeria monocytogenes* can cause listeriosis, with high fever, severe headache, neck stiffness, and nausea as its primary symptoms. In rare cases, listeriosis is fatal; it can also cause miscarriages and stillbirths. Pregnant women, the very young, elderly, and persons with compromised immune systems are the most susceptible. (FDA, 2018a).

1.2.2.2 Hong Lee Trading Inc. Issues Allergen Alert on Undeclared Milk Allergens in Chao Café Vietnamese Instant Coffee Mixed 3 in 1 (2018)

Hong Lee Trading Inc., New York, recalled its Chao Café Vietnamese Instant Coffee Mixed 3 In 1, 384 g containers coded June 6, 2018 due to it containing undeclared milk allergens. Consumers who are allergic to milk allergens may run the risk of serious or life-threatening allergic reactions if they consume this product (FDA, 2018a).

1.2.2.3 Evershing International Trading Company Recalls Frozen Shredded Coconut Because of Possible Health Risk (2018)

Evershing International Trading Company recalled its 16 ounce Coconut Tree Brand Frozen Shredded Coconut product because it had the potential to be contaminated with *Salmonella*, an organism which can cause serious and sometimes fatal infections in young children, frail or elderly people, and others with weakened immune system. Healthy persons infected with *Salmonella* often experience fever, diarrhea (which may be bloody), nausea, vomiting, and abdominal pain. In rare circumstances, infection with *Salmonella* can result in the organism getting in to the bloodstream and producing more severe illnesses such as arterial infections (i.e., infected aneurysms), endocarditis, and arthritis. No illnesses have been reported to date (FDA, 2018a).

1.2.2.4 T. Marzetti Company Voluntarily Recalls Frozen Biscuit Dough Packed under Various Brands Due to Potential *Listeria* Contamination (2018)

T. Marzetti Company recalled "Best By" dates of various products that were distributed in Alabama, Florida, Georgia, Indiana, Kentucky, Louisiana, North Carolina, Pennsylvania, South Carolina, Tennessee, Texas, and Virginia, because they may have the potential to be contaminated with *Listeria monocytogenes* (FDA, 2018a).

1.2.2.5 Nodine's Smokehouse Inc. Recalls Smoked Salmon 1.5 lb, 8 oz Packages Due to Possible *Listeria monocytogenes* Contamination (2017)

Nodine's Smokehouse, Inc. of Torrington, Connecticut recalled Smoked Salmon 1.5 lb, 8 oz packages. Lot numbers 40173 and 33173 because they have the potential to be contaminated with *Listeria monocytogenes* (FDA, 2018a).

1.2.2.6 Fresh Pak Inc. Recalls Lot-Specific Sliced Apple Products Because of Possible Health Risk (2017)

Fresh Pak Inc. of Detroit, Michigan announced a voluntary lot-specific recall of red/green apple slices. Jack Brown Produce, Inc. (supplier) requested Fresh Pak Inc. to perform a recall for the reason that they could have potentially been contaminated with *Listeria monocytogenes* (FDA, 2018a).

1.2.2.7 Piller's Fine Foods Recalls Ready-to-Eat Salami and Speck Products Due to Possible Salmonella Adulteration (2017)

Piller's Fine Foods, Waterloo, Canada, recalled approximately 1,076 pounds of ready-to-eat salami and speck products that may have been adulterated with *Salmonella*.

1.2.3 RECENT DRUG RECALLS

1.2.3.1 Compounded Injectables

PharMEDium Services, LLC recalled compounded injectables due to lack of sterility assurance in 2017 (FDA, 2018b).

1.2.3.2 Linezolid Injection

AuroMedics recalled Linezolid Injection due to particulate contamination (mold) in 2017 (FDA, 2018b).

1.2.3.3 Pantoprazole Sodium Injection

AuroMedics Pharma, LLC recalled Pantoprazole Sodium for Injection 40 mg per vial due to the presence of glass particles in 2017 (FDA, 2018b).

1.2.3.4 Alcohol Prep Pads

Pharmacist Choice (Simple Diagnostics) recalled Alcohol Prep Pads due to lack of sterility assurance in 2017 (FDA, 2018a).

1.2.3.5 Riomet® (MetFormin Hydrochloride Oral Solution)

Sun Pharmaceutical Industries, Ltd. Recalled Riomet® (Metformin Hydrochloride Oral Solution), 500 mg/5 mL in 2017 (FDA, 2018b).

1.2.3.6 Amiodarone HCl

Baxter International, Inc. recalled Amiodarone HCl due to the presence of particulate matter in 2017 (FDA, 2018b).

1.2.4 COMMENTS

While there are several recalls listed here, contamination events and disinfection issues are an ongoing concern in regulated industries. Many FDA-483 observations and warning letters are issued each year for not performing cleaning and disinfection procedures correctly, failure to disinfect, and the potential for microbiological contamination (21 CFR §211.113). Another common observation is lack of sterility assurance, but this can be a contamination issue and/or an issue with a lack of the appropriate documentation.

1.3 WHY THIS BOOK IS IMPORTANT

Science and technology are constantly evolving. There are cleaning agents and disinfection agents that were state of the art when you were in school that may be banned or significantly outdated today. Unless you work entirely in that area of science or technology you may not be aware of better or more efficacious methods. This book provides you with the important updates you need to ensure that you have state-of-the-art procedures and methods.

For example:

- A complete overview of disinfectants and how they work and are used is provided.
- It describes why you may wish to use preservatives and how to qualify the use of preservatives.
- There are concerns with the formation of biofilms. This data is up to date and will aid in preventing contamination risks.
- A variety of new technologies are presented that can provide significant benefits in both your disinfection procedures and decontamination procedures.
- Information is provided on various sterilization methods that can be used for both decontamination and sterilization.
- New categories of disinfectants and sterilants that can also be used which are safer on the surfaces being cleaned, e.g., not corrosive.

1.4 CONCLUSION

This book provides copious information on the methods and controls to employ to ensure that your disinfection and decontamination procedures are safe and efficacious for your products. The various discussions will provide you with invaluable information for your endeavors.

LITERATURE CITED

FDA (2018a) Food Safety.gov. Recent Recalls. Downloaded from: www.foodsafety.gov/recall s/recent/index.html. Downloaded on January 9, 2018.

FDA (2018b) Drug Recalls. Downloaded from: www.fda.gov/drugs/drugsafety/drugrecalls/ default.htm. Downloaded on January 9, 2018.

Moldenhauer, J. (2017) The New England Compounding Pharmacy Meningitis Outbreak Remembered. The IVT Network. Downloaded from: www.ivtnetwork.com/article/new -england-compounding-pharmacy-meningitis-outbreakremembered. Downloaded on January 9, 2018.

2 Disinfectants and Biocides

Tim Sandle

CONTENTS

2.1   INTRODUCTION

This chapter reviews the use of disinfectants and biocides in the pharmaceutical and healthcare sectors. These agents are essential for maintaining contamination control. While the clean space within which the manufacturing and dispensing of medicines takes place is invariably well-designed (through filtered air, maintaining pressure differentials, suitable air-change rates and so on), microbial risks arise from in-coming goods, water, and through the activities of personnel. For these reasons, the regular cleaning and disinfection of surfaces is required (1). In addition, processing equipment requires frequent cleaning and disinfection; and periodic disinfection may be required for water systems.

The focus of this chapter is on disinfectants used in cleanrooms and other controlled areas for surface disinfection, which is necessary for maintaining contamination control (2). The chapter considers the different types of chemicals that are available as disinfection agents; the process for their selection; their application; and how they are to be qualified through disinfectant efficacy testing. In doing so the chapter does not seek to regurgitate regulatory standards (these are sign-posted for the reader to explore); instead the chapter seeks to provide a practical approach, supported by scientific theory, for the use of disinfectants and biocides for the purposes of microbial contamination control for pharmaceuticals and healthcare facilities.

2.2   TERMS AND DEFINITIONS

A disinfectant is a chemical agent that can kill or inactivate vegetative microorganisms. When judged against an accepted standard, "disinfection" can relate to the reduction of a known population to a required level (such as a six-log reduction of more than one million cells). Disinfectants vary in their spectrum of activity, modes of action and efficacy. Some are bacteriostatic, where the ability of the bacterial population to grow is halted. Here the disinfectant can cause selective and reversible changes to cells by interacting with nucleic acids, inhibiting enzymes or permeating into the cell wall. Other disinfectants are bactericidal in that they destroy bacterial cells through different mechanisms including causing structural damage to the cell; autolysis; cell lysis and the leakage or coagulation of cytoplasm. Within these groupings the spectrum of activity varies with some disinfectants being effective against vegetative Gram-positive and Gram-negative microorganisms only while others are effective against fungi.

Some disinfectants are sporicidal in that they can cause the destruction of endo-spore-forming bacteria (these are the most difficult forms of microorganisms to eliminate from cleanroom surfaces) (3). However, a chemical agent does not have to be sporicidal in order to be classed as a "disinfectant" or as a "biocide". Thus disinfection commonly refers to an agent that can destroy or inhibit vegetative microorganisms. Most disinfectants also possess virucidal properties.

All disinfectants are biocides; biocide is an umbrella terms of antimicrobial agents. There is a difference in interpretation of the term biocide between the US and Europe. A biocide is defined by the European Union as a chemical substance intended to destroy, deter, render harmless, or exert a controlling effect on any harmful organism. In addition to chemical agents, biological substances are also classed as biocides (such as a fungus that would inhibit a bacterium) (4). The US Environmental Protection Agency (EPA) defines biocides as "a diverse group of poisonous substances including preservatives, insecticides, disinfectants, and pesticides used for the control of organisms that are harmful to human or animal health or that cause damage to natural or manufactured products" (5). Thus the EPA definition is somewhat wider, embracing plant protection products and some veterinary medicines. This is not a contextual problem for this chapter, where the focus is with disinfectants used in pharmaceutical and healthcare facilities.

2.3 KILLING, INACTIVATING, AND INHIBITING MICROORGANISMS

With a microbial cell there is a common sequence of events whereby the disinfectant interacts with the cell surface; this is followed by penetration into the cell and action at the target site(s) (6). Different disinfectants attack microbial cells in different ways; and, conversely, different species of microorganisms vary in their resistance to different disinfectants. These can be affected by the population of microorganisms present, their species, and the community with which they are bound.

One important determinant is with the numbers of organisms. A disinfection agent is considerably more effective against a low number of microorganisms than a higher number or a population with a greater cell density. Similarly, a disinfectant is more effective against a pure population than a mixed population of microorganisms. Use of a routine disinfectant will not be likely to kill all microorganisms present and a number will remain viable. Whether the surviving microorganisms multiply in sufficient number is dependent upon the condition in which the surviving population remains, the available nutrients, and the time between repeat applications of the disinfectant.

Following from numbers, different types of microorganisms have varying levels of resistance to broad spectrum disinfectants. This can be represented by the "classic" hierarchy of resistance, as shown in Figure 2.1. The increased resistance is primarily due to the cell membrane composition or type of protein coat.

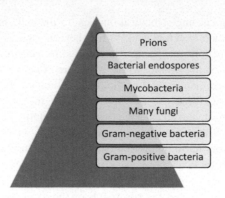

FIGURE 2.1   Pyramid of resistance to common disinfectants (adapted from Russell, 1986) (7).

Resistance is acquired through natural genetic properties of the microorganisms or it is acquired through phenotypic or genotypic variations (similar to antibiotic resistance through the overuse of one type of disinfectant). Generally, innate sensitivity results in Gram-negative bacteria being more resistant to disinfectant applications than Gram-positive bacteria. The reason for the increased resistance among Gram-negative bacteria can be attributed to a greater abundance of a hydrophobic lipopolysaccharides (LPS) in the cell membrane, whereas the Gram-positive membrane is primarily made up of inelastic "murein sacculi". It is interesting that within the group of least resistant, Gram-positive bacteria, there are microorganisms (e.g., *Bacillus*, *Clostridium*, etc.) that can produce endospores which are the several degrees more resistant than their vegetative counterpart. This may be because of the relative impermeability of the polypeptides which make up the spore coat to hydrophilic agents.

A final factor shaping resistance is with the location of the organisms. The location of microorganisms can influence the effectiveness of a disinfectant. Microorganisms in suspension are easier to kill than those affixed to surfaces. This is due to the mechanisms of microorganism attachment, such as bacteria fixing themselves using fimbriae or when a biofilm community develops (8). Such positioning impacts the contact time required for the disinfectant to bind to the microorganism, cross the cell wall, and act at the target site.

2.4   THE IMPORTANCE OF PRE-CLEANING

Ensuring that surfaces are regularly disinfected and that the numbers of bacteria present are kept to a minimum is of great importance. However, most disinfectants are only effective when used in conjunction with a detergent. This is because most disinfectants have poor cleaning ability and will not easily penetrate "soil" (dust, grease, and dirt). So surfaces must be rinsed frequently with a detergent and then disinfected at frequent intervals. Organic matter may reduce the activity of the disinfectant by either reacting chemically with the disinfectant or blocking the physical access of the disinfectant to the microbial target (9).

Detergents generally work by penetrating soil and reducing the surface tension (which adhere soil to the surface) to allow its removal (in crude terms, a detergent increases the "wettability" of water). Many detergents are synthetic "surfactants" (an acronym for Surface Active Agents).

Whilst "cleaning" is not "disinfection", the cleaning process can remove or dilute microbial populations. Nevertheless, the important distinction is that while disinfectants kill and inactivate microorganisms, detergents do not (although some detergents are formulated with antimicrobial chemicals). The purpose of a detergent is to clean and removal soil. The best detergents not only clean, they will be formulated as not to react with disinfectants where detergent residues remain on surfaces. Most compatible detergents are close to a neutral pH (10).

In selecting detergents, it is important that:

- The detergent is neutral and non-ionic solutions.
- The detergent should be non-foaming.
- The detergent should be compatible with the disinfectant (that is the residues of the detergent will not inactivate the disinfectant).

For aseptic processing areas, the detergent should also be sterile.

2.5   TYPES OF DISINFECTANTS

Disinfectants can be divided into two groups: non-oxidizing and oxidizing. Non-oxidizing disinfectants include alcohols (which disrupt the bacterial cell membranes); aldehydes (which denature bacterial cell proteins and can cause coagulation of cellular protein); amphoterics (which have both anionic and cationic character and possess a relative wide spectrum of activity); phenolics (some phenols cause bacterial cell damage through disruption of proton motive force); and quaternary ammonium compounds (QACs, which cause cytoplasm leakage and cytoplasm coagulation through interaction with phospholipids). QACs are among the most commonly used disinfectants (11).

Oxidizing agents have a wider spectrum of activity than non-oxidizing disinfectants and can damage endospores. However, they pose greater risks to human health. This group includes: halogens like iodine, peracetic acid and chlorine dioxide. For these "sporidical" disinfectants it is common to use the word "sporicide" to differentiate these agents from standard disinfectants.

2.5.1   COMMON NON-SPORICIDAL DISINFECTANTS

The majority of disinfectants outlined below have a specific mode of action against microorganisms and generally have a lower spectrum of activity compared to oxidizing disinfectants. The list is far from absolute; the intention is to describe the more common types of disinfectants found within the pharmaceutical or healthcare setting.

2.5.2   ALCOHOLS

Alcohols have an antibacterial action against vegetative cells. The effectiveness of alcohols against vegetative bacteria increases with their molecular weight (i.e., ethanol is more effective than methanol and in turn isopropyl alcohols are more effective than ethanol). Alcohols, where efficacy is increased with the presence of water, act on the bacterial cell wall by making it permeable. This can result in cytoplasm leakage, denaturation of protein and eventual cell lysis (alcohols are one of the so called "membrane disrupters"). The advantages of using alcohols include a relatively low cost, little odor and quick evaporation. However, alcohols have very poor action against bacterial and fungal spores and can only inhibit spore germination at best (12).

2.5.3 ALDEHYDES

Formaldehyde and gluteraldehyde are common to the aldehydes. Gluteraldehyde is a very effective disinfectant (and sterilant), has a wide spectrum of activity, and is effective against bacterial and fungal spores. However, gluteraldehyde is little used today due to personnel health and safety concerns. Formaldehyde and o-phthaladehyde are slightly less effective in comparison due to a slower rate of reaction, but possesses an equally wide spectrum of activity. Aldehydes have a non-specific effect in the denaturing of bacterial cell proteins and can cause coagulation of cellular protein (13).

2.5.4 AMPHOTERICS

Amphoterics are acidic and have a relative wide spectrum of activity, but are limited by their ability to damage bacterial endospores. An example is alkyl di(aminoethyl) glycine or derivatives (14).

2.5.5 ACID ANIONICS

Acid anionics are weak acids with a relatively limited spectrum of activity and are very pH dependent. An example of this group is carboxylic acid. They are not effective against fungi or spore-forming bacteria. Their bactericidal properties arise from their ability to cause cell disruption through proton motive force where the balance of hydrogen across the cell is disrupted which can affect cellular division by disruption of oxidative phosphorylation (15).

2.5.6 BIGUANIDES

Biguanides are polymers supplied in salt form, such as chlorhexidine, alexidine, and hydrochloride. Biguanides have a relatively wide spectrum of activity with the exception of killing bacterial endospores. This group is most effective at an alkaline pH and is rarely effective under acidic conditions. Biguanides affect the bacterial cell membrane and enter the cell through diffusion causing cell disruption and cytoplasm leakage (16).

2.5.7 PHENOLICS

Phenols are produced from the fractionation of tar and are among the oldest scientifically evaluated disinfectants, dating back to Robert Koch's evaluation of phenol's bactericidal effect against *Bacillus anthracis*. The commonly used phenolic is basic phenol (carbolic acid) although synthetic variants are widely used. Phenol can be made more complex by the addition of halogens such as chlorine (the bis-phenols and halophenols) to make compounds like triclosan and chloroxylenol. Phenols are bactericidal and antifungal, but are not effective against bacterial spores. Some phenols cause bacterial cell disruption through proton motive force while others attack the cell wall and cause leakage of cellular components and protein denaturation (17).

2.5.8 Quaternary Ammonium Compounds (QACs)

QACs are cationic salts of organically substituted ammonium compounds and have a fairly broad range of activity against microorganisms, although more effective against Gram-positive bacteria at lower concentrations than Gram-negative bacteria. They are considerably less effective against bacterial spores. QACs are sometimes classified as surfactants. An example is benzalkonium chloride (18). QACs are the most widely used of the non-oxidizing disinfectants in the pharmaceutical industry. Their mode of action is on the cell membrane which leads to cytoplasm leakage and cytoplasm coagulation through interaction with phospholipids (19).

2.5.9 Sporicidal Agents

Sporicidal agents are designed to render bacterial or fungal spores no longer able to germinate and produce viable, vegetative cells. This class of chemicals are typically powerful oxidizing agents which elicit their kill by the oxidation of proteins and other key cellular components (12). The types of chemicals used as agents include: ethylene oxide, glutaraldehyde, formaldehyde, hydrogen peroxide, peracetic acid, chlorine dioxide, sodium hypochlorite, sodium dichloroisocyanurate, and ozone- and iodine-based products (20, 21).

Sporicidal agents should not be confused with agents that are merely sporistatic agents. These chemicals act on bacterial spores via a different mechanism. Primarily they act and kill as the spore germinates back to a vegetative cell, but they do not kill the spore. Examples of these agents include biguanides, quaternary ammonium compounds, di- and tri-amines, and phenols (22).

The ideal sporicidal agent will effectively kill the following:

- Bacteria – Gram-positive and Gram-negative.
- Fungi including fungal spores, molds, and yeast.
- Enveloped and naked viruses (where required).
- Bacterial spores.

2.5.9.1 Examples of Sporicides

Some of the types of sporicidal agents, commonly found in the pharmaceutical and healthcare sectors are (23):

- Hypochlorous acid. This is a weak acid with the chemical formula HOCl. It forms when chlorine dissolves in water, and it is the HOCl moiety that actually does the disinfection. The chemical elicits its bactericidal activity

by acting on a wide variety of biomolecules, including DNA, RNA, fatty
acid groups, cholesterol, and proteins.

- Sodium dichloroisocyanurate (NaDCC). NaDCC is a chemical compound
widely used as a cleansing agent and disinfectant; this salt is an active
ingredient in many bleaches.
- Chlorine dioxide is a chemical compound with the formula ClO_2. As one of
several oxides of chlorine, it is a potent and useful oxidizing agent.
- Hypochlorites. This is a compound of chlorine and oxygen, with a chemical
formula ClO^-, which can combine with a number of counter ions such as
Na+ (household bleach) and Ca^+ (used for water treatment) ions, to form the
corresponding hypochlorites.
- Hydrogen peroxide (H_2O_2) is a colorless liquid that is the simplest peroxide
(a compound with an oxygen-oxygen bond). It is used as a strong oxidizer,
bleaching agent, and disinfectant.
- Peracetic acid (also referred to as peroxyacetic acid) is an organic compound with the formula CH_3CO_3H. It is a colorless liquid with a characteristic acrid odor similar to acetic acid (e.g., vinegar). Peracetic acid is often
combined with acetic acid or hydrogen peroxide in solution to maintain the
stability of the peracid.

2.5.10 HAND SANITIZATION

Personnel carry many types of microorganisms on their hands and such microorganisms can be readily transferred from person to person, or from person to
equipment or critical surfaces. Such microorganisms (including those that are
found on human skin like *Staphylococcus*, *Micrococcus*, and *Propionibacterium*)
are either present on the skin not multiplying (transient flora) or are multiplying
microorganisms released from the skin (residential flora) (24). For critical operations in pharmaceuticals and healthcare, some protection is afforded by wearing
gloves. However, gloves are not suitable for all activities and gloves, if not regularly sanitized or if they are of an unsuitable design, will pick up and transfer
contamination.

A distinction is sometimes drawn between antiseptics and hand sanitizers (25).
Antiseptics are antimicrobial substances that are applied topically (to living tissue or
to skin) in order to reduce the possibility of infection, sepsis, or putrefaction occurring. Antiseptics are different to sanitizers, which are applied to gloved hands. Often
the chemicals found in sanitizers are unsuitable for skin due to the types of chemicals used to formulate them.

Hand sanitizers fall into two groups: alcohol based, which are more common,
and non-alcohol based. The most commonly used alcohol-based hand sanitizers are isopropyl alcohol or some form of denatured ethanol (such as industrial methylated spirits), normally at a 70% concentration. The more common
non-alcohol-based sanitizers contain either chlorhexidine or hexachlorophene.
For hand sanitizers used on skin, these must not cause excessive drying and be
non-irritating.

2.6   WHAT DETERMINES DISINFECTION SUCCESS?

Whether a disinfectant is successful in the intended aim is based upon its appropriate selection (which will include whether the disinfectant has been shown, experimentally, to be effective through validation as discussed below). There are other influencing factors that can affect how well a disinfectant may or may not work. These are:

- Type and quantity of the organism, as this presents the specific level of challenge to the agent(s) and so the concentrations required.
- Amount of protein-based materials present as this tends to inactivate and absorb the disinfectant.
- Presence of other organic compounds and soaps (e.g. non-ionic surfactants) either in the solution or the surfaces, as these interact with certain disinfectants even neutralizing them. In certain combinations this could enhance the effect for example quaternary ammonium compounds. In order for a disinfectant to be effective it must come into contact with and be absorbed by the microbial cell. If substances, such as oil, dirt, paper, or grease, act as a spatial barrier between the microbial cell and the disinfectant, the efficacy of the disinfectant will be adversely affected. The presence of such substances ("soil") halts disinfectant efficacy by either reacting with the disinfectant or creating a barrier for the disinfectant. This effect is increased if the surface itself has defects and crevices which limit disinfectant penetration.
- The solution will also be affected by other inherent characteristics namely pH, temperature, concentration, and possible interactions between other agents and containers. Generally, temperature influences the rate of reaction (26). Most disinfectants are more effective and kill a population faster at higher temperatures although many disinfectants, due to practical considerations, are manufactured to be used at ambient. Some disinfectants, particularly oxidizing agents like peracetic acid, have an optimal temperature of 40–50°C, and sporicidal agents like o-phthaladehyde are more effective at temperatures elevated above ambient. Disinfectants which are sensitive to temperatures other than ambient are normally assessed through the use of a temperature coefficient, or Q10 (which relates the increase in activity to a 10°C rise in temperature).
- The effect of pH is important because it influences the ionic binding of a disinfectant to a bacterial cell wall thereby ensuring disinfectant molecules bind to a high number of microorganisms. Many disinfectants are more stable at a set pH range, for example, acid-based disinfectants can become less potent in alkaline conditions whereas a gluteraldehyde is more potent at a basic pH. The use of a disinfectant outside of its desired pH range results in reduced efficacy.

2.7   SELECTION CRITERIA

The optimal requirements for a disinfectant include (27):

- A disinfectant must have a wide spectrum of activity. This refers to the ability of the disinfectant to kill different types of microorganisms and microorganisms which are in different physiological states.

- Where two disinfectants are used the disinfectants selected must have different modes of action.
- Rapid action, with contact times no longer than five minutes and ideally less than two minutes. The contact time is the time taken for the disinfectant to bind to the microorganism, traverse the cell wall and membrane, and to reach its specific target site. The longer the contact time, then the longer the surface needs to be left for prior to use. For the contact time the surface needs to remain "wet".
- Effective penetration, including being able to penetrate biofilms and remaining effective with general levels of soiling.
- Being chemically stable throughout its allocated shelf life and effective shelf life once opened.
- Durability, that is effective for the full period of contact (for this the disinfectant should remain wet and not degrade).
- Be compatible with materials; if there is a risk of corrosion, surfaces should be wiped with water or 70% IPA.

To the above, health and safety is an additional important requirement. The impact of handling many disinfectant products on the health and safety of the operatives needs to be considered. Many agents, like chlorine, hydrogen peroxide and peracetic acid are each potentially hazardous (28). Here the method of application is the main risk determinant (that is, spraying presents a higher risk to the operative compared to wiping as a result of a higher exposure to the operative). Many disinfectant products are generally irritants, in particular to the mucous membranes. Additionally, they are irritants to the eyes, respiratory tract, and skin; having differing effects depending on concentration and accessibility. This means a health and safety risk assessment should be conducted (assessing occupational exposure limits) and operators equipped with appropriate personal protective clothing (29).

2.8   DISINFECTANT FORMATS

The presentation of the disinfectant is an important choice, whether as a pre-diluted preparation in a trigger spray or as a ready-to-use concentrate or an impregnated wipe. These three common formats, together with some advantages and disadvantages, are considered next.

2.8.1   CONCENTRATES

The advantages of using concentrates over the ready prepared solution include ease of storage and the ability to vary the concentration according to needs. There is however a problem of the concentrates being quite corrosive and if not dissolved evenly can lead to ineffective disinfection.

2.8.2   SPRAY BOTTLES

Some spray bottles are poorly designed and allow for ingress of contamination into the reservoir of the bottle during use due to sucking back. One solution to the problem has been to introduce a collapsible bag inside the bottle which stops any vacuum being created and drawing back potentially contaminated air to come in contact with the solution. The manufacturer should produce efficacy data show the effectiveness of the spray mechanism for any disinfectant spray format purchased.

2.8.3 WIPES

The purpose of wipes is to:

- physically remove the bioburden from the surface;
- ensure the presence of sufficient disinfectant for long enough to kill vegetative and where possible, spore forming microorganisms;
- facilitate the destruction and removal of contaminants by the application of pressure against microbial cell walls during the wiping process.

With disinfectant wipes, impregnated wipes appear to demonstrate a greater reduction in bioburden than dry wipes which are wetted *in situ*. This is perhaps because dry wipes are rarely wetted enough to readily release sufficient alcohol onto the surface. In addition, the undulating and micro-structures of surfaces being disinfected does not always facilitate the effective delivery of disinfectant by the wipe process (30).

A further factor to consider with wipes is the material used to manufacture the wipe. This relates to particle deposition and degree of "wipability". Natural fiber wipes potentially shed more particulates; however, they tend to perform better than most synthetic materials, holding more liquid and therefore releasing more disinfectant to kill surface-borne organisms. These types of wipes also entrap particles and absorb residues more readily. Synthetic wipes (commonly fashioned from a polyester and cellulose mix) are low particle generating because, with the higher quality wipes, they are laser edged sealed in order to reduce fraying at the edges and any particle generation. The material selected must be inert to the agent for the shelf life of the product. Hypochlorites are known to react with polycellulose wipes over time so the chemical agent would be less effective over time.

2.9 DISINFECTANT ROTATION

When cleanroom disinfectants are selected many users opt to select two or more disinfectants. This is can be for several reasons (31):

- Most disinfectants do not have a complete spectrum of activity effective against all microorganisms (*spectrum of activity* is the ability of the disinfectant to kill different types of microorganisms and microorganisms which are in different physiological states) (32). The disinfectants commonly used are often effective against vegetative cells but are not sporicidal. To maintain an effective contamination control, the elimination of bacterial endospores through a sporicidal disinfectant is recommended (these are sometimes referred to as high-level disinfectants). Here a sporicide would be used in rotation with a non-sporicidal disinfectant.

- The disinfectants with the formulations which are effective against the greatest range of microorganisms are often expensive. With this, many manufacturers use a general broad spectrum disinfectant daily or weekly with a sporicidal disinfectant used weekly or monthly (a decision often based on the results of microbiological environmental monitoring and the characterization of the isolated microorganisms).
- Some disinfectants, such as sporicides, are corrosive. While the risk to surfaces can be reduced through rinsing, rotation is sometimes undertaken in order to reduce the risk of damage to cleanroom equipment and working benches.
- Some regulatory authorities, including the European Medicines Agency and the UK MHRA, require two disinfectants to be used in rotation which is a good manufacturing practice (GMP) requirement. The argument for rotating two disinfectants is to reduce the possibility of resistant strains of microorganisms developing. Whilst the phenomenon of microbial resistance is an issue of major concern for antibiotics there are few data to support development of resistance to disinfectants (33). Nonetheless, it remains a regulatory expectation.

Thus, the reasons for rotation are approached from either a desire to widen the mode of action or to address anticipated regulatory concerns.

2.10 APPLICATION OF DISINFECTANTS

The way that disinfectants are applied to surfaces can have a significant impact on the effectiveness of the disinfection process (34). Factors of importance include the materials used and the techniques applied. This section considers some good practice examples.

2.10.1 CLEANING AND DISINFECTION SCHEDULES

The facility needs to consider how often to clean and disinfect. This should be based upon a field trial and regular reviews of environmental monitoring (see below). With this information, cleaning and disinfection schedules can be constructed. Clear instructions must be provided for the cleaning and disinfection schedule to be followed for the cleanroom facility and the documentation to be completed to record the cleaning undertaken. This may reference a series of work instructions that provide step-by-step instructions for the cleaning of the cleanroom facility and its equipment. The applied frequencies and areas of application are best determined by risk assessment.

This risk assessment is performed to document the risks to product quality presented by sources of contamination and to identify the potential transfer route of this contamination. The document assesses the risk and the effect of steps taken to mitigate and minimize this risk. In a typical risk assessment, cleaning procedures will be used to mitigate many of the risks like the contamination of surfaces by people, material transfer, air movements, and so on.

One common approach is to classify the facility into three areas:

- Critical areas (i.e., production areas or directly adjacent, e.g., operations room, cryo-storage room).
- General areas (i.e., areas which are in the cleanroom facility and are maintained by with a low particulate count by the air handling regime, e.g., change rooms, consumables cupboards).
- Other areas (i.e., areas which are outside the primary facility e.g., bulk store rooms, cold store rooms which are not maintained in the same air handling regime).

Surfaces in each of the three areas will be cleaned at different frequencies depending upon their proximity to the critical areas and the ease of dispersion or transfer of contaminants.

2.10.2 Mops and Wipes

The common application of a disinfectant to a surface is either via a wipe (pre-saturated or where a disinfectant is sprayed and then wiped) or via a mop. A mop may either have a saturated wipe fitted to it (as with a single-use system), or the mop is plunged into a bucket. The material of the mop head is important. Mop head materials need to be able to abrasive enough to remove contamination and be robust enough to deal with much greater surface areas and the potential to transfer large quantities of cleaning agents to them quickly. Dry wipe heads can be as simple multilayer wipe that can be attached to an appropriate mop tool. They may have a light foam layer bound to them to allow for maintaining contact over uneven surfaces. Alternatives to this are microfiber heads that are electrostatically charged to attract and hold particles in during cleaning.

The greater part of mop heads for use with disinfectants are constructed using a polyester wipe bound to a much larger inner core of polyurethane foam. The foam gives the absorbance and the greater the amount of foam the larger the fluid capacity of the mop system. Some heads may just have the polyurethane foam, but these are prone to damage and snagging when moved over uneven surfaces.

2.10.3 Double or Triple Bucket System

Where mops are put into liquid disinfectant, good cleanroom practices typically dictate that a double or triple bucket system is used. With a two-bucket system the bucket next to the ringer would contain water to rinse the mop head once soiled. The head should be rung through before being placed in the disinfectant containing bucket and then placed in the ringer again before cleaning surfaces again. Excess solution would increase the drying time. A three-bucket system involves rinsing in the middle bucket and rear bucket is empty so when the mop is rung that waste solution does not cross-contaminate the rinsing or disinfectant containing buckets. When rinsing the mop heads is rinsed care must be taken to ensure that the head does no touch the bottom of the bucket. Particulate contaminants would settle at the bottom of the bucket and making contact would pick them up.

To summarize the steps more succinctly:

Two-Bucket Technique
1. Dip the mop in the disinfectant.
2. Mop the floor (preferably a specified number of square meters per "dipping").
3. Dip the mop in the bucket of water.
4. Rinse the excess water off the mop head back into the bucket of water (this is to prevent carrying too much water back into the disinfectant and diluting it).
5. Dip the mop in disinfectant.
6. Repeat.

Three-Bucket Technique
1. Dip the mop in disinfectant.
2. Mop the floor.
3. Dip the mop in the bucket of water.
4. Rinse the excess water off the mop head into the third (empty) bucket.
5. Dip the mop in disinfectant.
6. Repeat.

2.10.4 CLEANING AND DISINFECTION TECHNIQUES

Different parts of the facility will require cleaning and disinfection in different ways. Taking floors as an example, a model approach for floor cleaning or disinfection would be (35):

1. Either roll all of the floor surface with a tacky roller to remove any loose debris and fibers, moving any equipment to one half of the room nearest exit door, or wipe the floor using a neutral detergent solution and mop and bucket.
2. Use a use disinfectant impregnated mop wipes and mops (alternatively a mop with a ready prepared disinfectant solution could be used).
3. Using overlapping mop strokes, wipe down half the floor area, working methodically around the area starting at furthest reach point and working toward yourself in a straight line. Replace the mop wipe if the wipe becomes visibly contaminated or dry.
4. NOTE: Particular attention should be paid to corners and edges.
5. Leave the disinfectant solution on the surface for the manufacturer's recommended contact time to allow the disinfectant to be effective.
6. Remove the mop head and discard to waste.
7. Fit a second mop head with ethanol impregnated mop wipe (alternatively a mop with a ready prepared alcohol solution could be used).
8. After the allotted time, using the fresh mop head wipe down using overlapping mop strokes to remove any residue, working methodically around the area starting at furthest reach point and working toward yourself in a straight line. Replace the mop wipe if the wipe becomes visibly contaminated or dry.

9. Move equipment to cleaned floor area ensuring that contact surfaces are wiped prior to being replaced on clean surface.

10. Repeat steps for other half of floor area.

2.10.5 RINSING DISINFECTANT RESIDUES

Some disinfectants leave residues on surfaces. Whilst this can mean a continuation of an antimicrobial activity, residues can also lead to sticky surfaces and or the inactivation of other disinfectants. In such circumstances rinsing should take place using either water or alcohol. The type of water used will depend on the cleanroom grade (for example, purified water is suitable for non-sterile pharmaceutical facilities whereas sterile water-for-injection should be used for aseptic processing areas) (36).

2.10.6 DISPOSAL OF AGENTS

After any cleaning or disinfectant activity it is important to dispose of waste materials in waste bags and seal. Waste bags should be removed from the cleanroom suite via waste hatches. The bags should be disposed of in accordance with appropriate facility waste management procedures. In terms of cleaning solutions, local regulations should be adhered to. If these permit disposal down a drain, this should be accompanied with copious amounts of water.

2.10.7 STERILE DISINFECTANTS

Certain high-grade cleanroom activities require disinfectants to be sterile (such as aseptic preparation areas). For this, disinfectants can be purchased which have been sterile-filtered (through a 0.2 μm filter) and are provided in gamma-irradiated containers with outer wrapping.

2.10.8 HAND SANITIZERS AND ANTISEPTICS

There are a number of practical steps which need to be considered when using antiseptics and sanitizers within a healthcare or pharmaceutical facility. For disinfecting hands, hands should be washed using soap and water for around twenty seconds. Handwashing removes around 99% of transient microorganisms (although it does not kill them) (37). From then on, whether gloves are worn or not, regular hygienic hand disinfection should take place to eliminate any subsequent transient flora and to reduce the risk of the contamination arising from resident skin flora.

With gloved hands, the technique of hand sanitization is of great importance as the effectivity is not only with the antiseptic but also relates to the "rub-in" technique. For example:

Dispense a small amount of hand gel onto the palm of one hand, put hands together and proceed to rub the antiseptic into both hands. Pay particular attention to the following areas:

- Fingernails
- Back of hands

- Wrists
- Between webs of fingers
- Thumb

Allow hands to dry; this should take no more than 60 seconds.

Regular applications of hand sanitizer are required prior to carrying out critical activities. This is because alcohols are relatively volatile and do not provide a continual antimicrobial action.

2.10.9   OTHER GOOD PRACTICES

Other good practices for the adoption and use of disinfectants are:

- Written procedures should be in place.
- Responsibilities for cleaning should be assigned. Often this is interpreted as the need to have independent cleaning staff separate from those involved in product manufacture.
- Staff must be trained in cleaning techniques and have a training record.
- Details of cleaning frequencies, methods, equipment, and materials must be recorded in written procedures (Code of Federal Regulations [CFR]). This may relate to an approved supplier specification.
- The cleaning of equipment and materials must take place at regular intervals.
- Inspection of equipment for cleanliness before use should be part of routine operations.
- A cleaning log should be kept. The purpose is to keep a record of the areas cleaned, agents used, and the identity of the operator.
- The microorganisms isolated (the microbiota) from environmental monitoring programs should be examined for resistant strains. Some isolates from these reviews should be incorporated into disinfectant efficacy studies.
- The monitoring for microbial contamination in disinfectant and detergent solutions should be periodically undertaken.
- The storing of disinfectant and detergent solutions should be for defined (and short) periods.
- Room use should be recorded after each operation.
- There should be a technical agreement with the company who supplies the disinfectant. Ideally the disinfectants purchased should be lot tracked.

2.11   DISINFECTANT EFFICACY TESTING

It is a regulatory expectation that disinfectants used in controlled environments and cleanrooms have undergone a qualification by the facility. This is because the testing performed by the manufacturer of the disinfectant is typically only in the form of a basic suspension test and this level of testing does not take into account the different variables of use, including method of preparation, application, different surfaces, and so forth.

The regulatory expectations can be evidenced from the following documents:

PIC/S PI 007-6 – Recommendation on the Validation of Aseptic Processes (38): "The effectiveness of disinfectants and the minimum contact time on different surfaces should be validated."

FDA Guidance for Industry – Sterile Drug Products Produced by Aseptic Processing, Current Good Manufacturing Practice (39): "The suitability, efficacy, and limitations of disinfecting agents and procedures should be assessed. The effectiveness of these disinfectants and procedures should be measured by their ability to ensure that potential contaminants are adequately removed from surfaces."

The purpose of the main part of disinfectant tests is that they should simulate, as closely as possible in the laboratory, the in-use conditions that the disinfectants would be subjected to in practical use. Disinfectant efficacy tests are not easy to perform, and the analyst will need proven skills in the preparing and pipetting microbial cultures in a reliable and reproducible way (40).

There are two primary standards bodies that describe disinfectant efficacy tests: AOAC International, which includes carrier tests (surface tests) and use-dilution tests (suspension tests) for bactericidal, mycobactericidal, sporicidal, fungicidal, and virucidal activity; and the CEN (European Committee for Normalization), for the European Union, which includes a similar array of tests (as three phases) albeit with subtle differences (41). To these, the ASTM E2614-08 Guide for Evaluation of Cleanroom Disinfectants is also useful (which identifies important factors to consider when selecting a disinfectant for use in a cleanroom or similar controlled environment and recommends test methods suitable for evaluating disinfectants) (42); as is the USP <1072> chapter (which is discussed below). The differences in execution are not dissected in this chapter, although the broad differences between suspension tests, surface tests, and field trials are outlined.

2.11.1 APPROACHING DISINFECTANT VALIDATION

There are different approaches that can be taken for disinfectant validation. A common approach, and one of the most straightforward, is summarized in the United States Pharmacopeia. Chapter USP <1072> "Antiseptics and Disinfectants" (43) states:

> To demonstrate the efficacy of a disinfectant…it may be deemed necessary to conduct the following tests:
>
> 1. In-use dilution tests
> 2. Surface challenge tests
> 3. A statistical comparison of the frequency of isolation and numbers of microorganisms isolated prior to and after the implementation of a new disinfectant.

Both suspension tests and surface tests are conducted under clean and "dirty" conditions. Clean conditions are intended to cover applications where the surfaces can be cleaned sufficiently before the application of the disinfectant, whilst dirty conditions are intended to cover applications where cleaning prior to disinfection is not undertaken or cannot be relied upon to produce a clean surface. On this basis, the simulated dirty conditions are arguably more important. Suspension and surface tests are divided between tests for vegetative bacteria, test for fungi, and tests for bacterial spores (44).

The in-use (or suspension test) involves taking the disinfectant, at the required concentration, and adding to it an interfering substance (to simulate practical conditions) together with a known concentration of a challenge microorganism (derived from an 18–24-hour culture). The suspension is then held for the required contact time and at a defined temperature. Once this time has elapsed, a proportion of the challenged disinfectant is transferred to a tube containing a suitable neutralizer, which is intended to inactive the disinfectant. Once sufficient time has been given for neutralization, microbial survivors are assessed by plating out or filtering the disinfectant-neutralizer solution using a microbial culture method.

It is important that the neutralizer used has been tested in advance to show that it is not toxic to any microbial survivors. An approach from this was outlined by Sutton and colleagues (45). This involves calculating both neutralizer efficacy ratios, by comparing the recovery of identical inocula from the neutralizing solution in the presence, or the absence, of a 1:10 dilution of the biocide; and neutralizer toxicity ratios, which are determined between recovery of viable microorganisms incubated for a short period in peptone, and in the neutralizing medium without the biocide. An effective and non-toxic neutralizer was established by ratios of ≥ 0.75.

Surface testing involves aliquoting onto a surface coupon a mix of the challenge organism and, where required, an interfering substance (such a protein, to simulate dirty conditions). The surface coupon will be fashioned from a representative surface in the cleanroom (here several different materials will require testing in order to show how the disinfectant performs). To this an amount of the test disinfectant is added. The solutions are left for the required contact time. Once the contact time has elapsed, the coupon is transferred to a neutralizer solution. Then, as with the suspension test once sufficient time has been given for neutralization, microbial survivors are assessed by plating out or filtering the disinfectant-neutralizer solution using a microbial culture method.

A possible array of surfaces to consider (this will be facility dependent) are:

- Stainless steel
- Glass
- Aluminum
- Epoxy
- Enamel
- Acrylic
- Mipolam
- Vinyl
- Hardwood
- Plastic
- Plexiglas
- Chromium

The statistical comparison part is commonly referred to as a field trial (*in situ* testing). This tests how well the disinfectant performs (either solely or in conjunction with another disinfectant in rotation) in the actual area(s) where the disinfectant will be used. The assessment is through surface-based environmental monitoring where microbial counts and species are assessed prior to and after the application of the disinfectant.

To run an effective field trial, a baseline is established prior to and then during implementation of the new regime using intensive environmental sampling. The effectiveness of the new disinfectant is accessed via a statistical evaluation of the environmental monitoring data before and after implementation of the new regime. The obtained results should be equivalent or better.

With the above three-step approach, some users elect to run in-use dilution tests (or suspension tests); others chose to conduct surface tests only; and some will conduct both.

2.11.2 SUSPENSION OR SURFACE TESTING?

One research study suggests that simply testing disinfectant efficacy for organisms in suspension is unrealistic when it comes to assessing the microbial inactivating properties of microorganisms found to surfaces, especially when the microorganisms are in biofilm communities (46). Microorganisms in suspension bacteria are easily eradicated in the test because they are readily exposed to disinfectants (47). To fully understand the ability of a disinfectant to destroy microorganisms surface studies are required. Therefore, to fully understand the disinfectant, surface testing must form a major part of any qualification study.

2.11.3 SELECTION OF THE MICROBIAL TEST PANEL AND ASSESSING MICROBIAL KILL

Many of the standards for disinfectant validation list a range of organisms; not all of these organisms will be appropriate for the life science sector. This is because the standards are written to cover a range of industries, including the food and veterinary sectors. It is important to demonstrate that the disinfectants used in pharmaceuticals and healthcare are effective against standard microorganisms applicable to this sector and commonly encountered environmental isolates on the predominant surfaces in the cleanroom. With the inclusion of environmental isolates (or "plant isolates"), this is a commonly requested item from regulators.

With typical organisms for an industrial facility (read "pharmaceutical facility"), the European series of disinfectant tests recommend the following bacteria:

- *Staphylococcus aureus* (American Type Culture Collection [ATCC] 6538)
- *Enterococcus hirae* (ATCC 10541)
- *Pseudomonas aeruginosa* (ATCC 15442)
- *Escherichia coli* (ATCC 10536)

And the following fungi:

- *Candida albicans* (ATCC 10231)
- *Aspergillus brasiliensis* (ATCC 16404)

With fungi it is recommended that fungal spores are used since the presence of hyphae and mycelia can prevent disinfectant from contacting and penetrating spores.

To assess a sporicidal disinfectant, the following organism as a spore suspension is recommended:

*   *Bacillus subtilis* (ATCC 6633)

Where virucidal properties are required:

*   Adenovirus-5 and poliovirus

(The virucidal assessment of disinfectants is outside the scope of this chapter).

Microbial kill is assessed through logarithmic reduction (as expressed to base 10). Log reductions are a relative concept and the log reduction obtained will be impacted by the starting inoculum. Take two examples, both of which lead to the same log reduction:

Test 1:

*   Test inoculum: 1×10^7 CFU
*   Survivors: 1×10^5 CFU
*   Log reduction: 2 log
*   Organisms killed: 9.9×10^6 CFU

Test 2:

*   Test inoculum: 1×10^5 CFU
*   Survivors: 1×10^3 CFU
*   Log reduction: 2 log
*   Organisms killed: 9.9×10^4 CFU

2.11.4 THE VALIDATION APPROACH

An approach that can be adopted for the validation of disinfectants to be used within the cleanroom is (48):

1. Screening tests. These may be used to compare various disinfectants (or different concentrations of a disinfectant) when making the choice of which disinfectants to purchase. This is usually by suspension testing.
2. Surface challenge tests. This is the most important disinfectant efficacy test and, as discussed above, typically conducted using standard organisms and environmental isolates on cleanroom surfaces.
3. Qualification of the environmental monitoring media for use in conjunction with chosen disinfectant (see below).
4. Field trial. The field trial is conducted after the laboratory-based assays have been completed. The field trials test whether the selected disinfectants work in practice. This is a study of organisms isolated (frequency and type)

before and after implementation of a new cleaning and disinfection regime. A field trial can also help to set appropriate frequencies of disinfection and the interval between the rotation of two different disinfectants.

There are several important factors that require assessing through disinfectant validation. These are (49):

- The concentration of the disinfectant. Many users will test the manufacturer's recommended concentration, which keeps this part more straightforward. However, if the user seeks to establish a concentration this needs to be added, including a minimum and maximum range. Setting the concentration is easier to establish through suspension tests.
- The contact time. This is time needed for the required level of microbial kill (or inactivation) to be achieved. A disinfectant product may have different contact times depending on the target organisms (for example an extended contact time will probably be needed for sporicidal action). In setting contact times it is important that these are practical; many standards set contact times that are unrealistically long (such as the European standard for sporidical efficacy – EN 13704 – which comes in at sixty minutes). A second area with contact times that needs to be factored in is the rate of drying. In the laboratory setting, disinfectants will dry more slowly than in the cleanroom (where the air-change rates are faster and the air is most likely to be less humid).
- The microbial challenge. Many disinfectant efficacy standards use very high challenges (up to one million microbial cells) and associated multi-step logarithmic reductions. These are far in excess of what would be found in a cleanroom. Lower challenges can be used, with justification. This can lead to more practical contact times, especially when assessing sporicidal agents. A two-log reduction, for example, of bacterial spores should be sufficient for most cleanrooms.
  An argument for accepting a lower log-kill acceptance criteria can be based on:
  - The case that disinfectants are less effective against the high numbers of organisms used during testing than against the low numbers expected in a cleanroom environment.
  - Stressed environmental organisms are easier to kill than the cultures using in testing.
  - In practical situations disinfectants are applied by wiping/moping which physically removes organisms enhancing the "kill".
- The types of surfaces. For surface testing a range of surfaces need to be tested. This will include common surfaces like vinyl, acrylic, glass, and laminate. Moreover, the surface type and condition can have a significant impact on efficacy (older or damaged surfaces can be more challenging).
- The quality of water used to dilute the disinfectant concentrate. The water quality (potable, purified, or water-for-injections) should be the same as used in the production facility.

- The temperature of use. Laboratory studies are commonly conducted at 20–25°C. This normally matches process conditions. However, consideration will need to be given if the disinfectant is intended to be used in cold rooms, for example, since these lower temperatures may affect disinfectant efficacy.

2.11.5 ADDITIONAL TESTING

Outside of the formal requirements of the standards, many users elect to conduct the following additional assessments:

a. Testing at the end of the shelf life of the product:
   1. Either as the solution *per se*,
   2. Or a solution in contact with either the synthetic or natural fiber wipe.
b. When a product is reconstituted:
   1. Just before use,
   2. And at the end of its in-use shelf life.

The reason for doing so particularly applies to sporicides, which are chemicals that are generally reactive oxidizing species. These chemicals are essentially unstable or reactive toward packaging or wipe materials.

In some cases, with the development of a novel agent, pre-studies may be performed for establishing the appropriate concentration. For this dilution methods can be used to establish the minimum inhibitory concentrations (MICs) of antimicrobial agents: these are the reference methods for antimicrobial susceptibility testing and are mainly used to establish the activity of a new agent, to confirm the susceptibility of microorganisms to the agent that give equivocal results in routine tests, and to determine the susceptibility on various microorganisms where routine tests may be unreliable (50). Other alternate procedures for assessing disinfectant effectiveness include flow cytometry (using cytofluorometry) (51).

2.11.6 REVALIDATION

Disinfectant validation is normally a one-time activity; this is reflective of the amount of resources required to run a study and the "self-validating" aspect which arises through regular reviews of the environmental monitoring data. Times may arise, however, when revalidation needs to be considered. Examples are:

- A significant change in the number and/or type of microorganisms identified (efficacy of current biocides against any new predominant organisms should be established).
- Change to the predominant surface types in the cleanroom: e.g., refurbishment, new equipment (efficacy of current biocides on new surfaces should be established).
- Change to the formulation of the biocide (requirement for full revalidation should be considered).

2.11.7 REGULATORY CONCERNS

Citations against improperly executed disinfectant studies are a common feature in FDA warning letters (along with mentions of no disinfectant efficacy data being available at all). Some common findings include:

- "No data to support the appropriateness of the disinfectants used..."
- "Did not include efficacy studies for solutions currently used..."
- "Did not use materials found in the aseptic processing area (APA) floors, walls, work surfaces..."
- "No data to support the expiration date..."
- "No data to support the contact time..."
- "The coupons used in the 'Disinfectant Efficacy Verification for Hard Surfaces'... were not representative of the surfaces found..."
- "Your disinfectant qualification for____ disinfectants documented that the log reduction criteria (Bacteria >4, Fungi >3) was not met when challenged with multiple organisms in variety of surfaces..."
- "There is no assurance that the disinfectant ____ is effective against mold, since it did not meet your established recovery rate acceptance criterion..."

These concerns are addressed in the preceding section provided a good disinfectant study design is written in advance of conducting validation runs.

2.12 ENVIRONMENTAL MONITORING

It is important that residual disinfectants on cleanroom surfaces do not interfere with the recovery of organisms from contact plates. This matters for the field trial and for the ongoing assessment of cleanrooms as part of the routine environmental monitoring program. This is overcome through the inclusion of a disinfectant neutralizer in the agar used for the contact plates used for surface sampling. Where there is a requirement to take finger dabs from the gloves worn by personnel (as is the case in sterile manufacturing environments), the agar plates used should also contain a neutralizer to guard against the risk of false negatives being recorded.

The results from environmental monitoring, as discussed above, can inform the effectiveness of the cleaning and disinfection program. This relates to assessing microbial numbers and species types. Regularly reoccurring species can be considered for inclusion in disinfectant efficacy tests (52).

2.13 ALTERNATIVES TO DISINFECTANT PRACTICES

Any disinfection practice, especially the transfer of items into and out of critical areas (so-termed "transfer disinfection") carries risks. The use of single-use sterile disposable items, which are wrapped in two or more layers of sterile wrapping, provide lower risk alternatives and, for sterile manufacturing at least, provide a lower-risk alternative. The use of terminal gamma-irradiated or ethylene oxide sterilized components offers an alternative to the use of liquid disinfection agents.

2.14   CLEANING VALIDATION

Pharmaceutical manufacturing involves both chemical and physical processes which take place through a series of multiple step processes. These processes involve a range of different items of equipment, from centrifuges through to ultrafiltration units. If cleaning procedures for such equipment, whether these be automated or manual, can give rise to contamination. The biggest risk is that such contamination remains in place by the time the next batch is manufactured. The types of contamination which may be present can include microorganisms; residues of previous products; other active pharmaceutical ingredients; cleaning agents; solvents or lubricants. The presence of residues creates problems for the elimination of microorganisms due to the properties of bacterial adhesion altering; for this reason, hold times need to be assessed (53).

To guard against these events, equipment needs to be subjected to cleaning validation. This is a specialist area which falls outside the direct scope of this chapter; it is mentioned here in order for completeness and to show the range of cleaning and disinfection practices in pharmaceutical and healthcare settings.

2.15   CONCLUSION

This chapter has provided an overview of the key considerations for the selection and use of disinfectants and biocides for pharmaceutical and healthcare facilities. As the text has shown, in order to achieve microbial control in cleanrooms and in other areas where the minimization of contamination is important, like laboratories, the use of defined cleaning techniques, together with the application of detergents and disinfectants, is of great importance. From the good manufacturing practices (GMP) perspective, the use of such detergents and disinfectants is a step toward control of contamination however the use of cleaning solutions should not merely cover up poor practices. Facility performance is also the product of the design, personnel practices, process and product controls, and control of incoming items. Disinfection supports these other control measures.

With using disinfectants, a number of important choices need to be made in terms of selection; using disinfectants in rotation; and in setting appropriate frequencies of application. These have been discussed in this chapter. Central to the choices made is validation, since the validation activity reveals significant information about the way the disinfectant works and its likely success in operation.

With disinfectant validation, the key messages are that before purchasing a new disinfectant the use should ensure that the minimum test criteria have been met by suppliers. The user should then, as regulators expect, perform their own validation. However, in doing so, a number of choices need to be made about the methods and acceptance criteria. In selecting these, the surface test is of more importance than the suspension test and once laboratory tests have been completed, the disinfectant requires testing in the cleanroom setting through extensive environmental monitoring.

The chapter has addressed these themes and, in presenting a practical series of steps to be reviewed, backed by scientific principles, it provides a framework for facilities to adopt or with which to assess their practices against.

REFERENCES

1. Sandle, T. (2012). Cleaning and disinfection. In Sandle, T. (Ed.) *The CDC Handbook: A Guide to Cleaning and Disinfecting Cleanrooms*, Grosvenor House Publishing: Surrey, UK, pp 1–31.
2. Sandle, T. and Vijaykumar, R. (2014) *Cleanroom Microbiology*, DHI/PDA: River Grove, USA, pp 369–374.
3. Sandle, T. (2016) Risk of microbial spores, prevention measures and disinfection strategies. In Madsen, R. E. and Moldenhaurer, J. (Eds.) *Contamination Control in Healthcare Product Manufacturing*, Volume 4, DHI: River Grove, USA, pp 59–95.
4. Biocidal Product Regulation (BPR, Regulation (EU) 528/2012), European Commission. Brussels, Belgium.
5. EPA. Product Performance Test Guidelines. OPPTS 810.1000 Overview, Definitions, and General Considerations, EPA 712–C–98–001, March 1998.
6. Brown, M. R. W. and Gilbert, P. (1993) Sensitivity of biofilms to antimicrobial agents. *Journal of Applied Bacteriology – Symposium Supplement*, 74: 87S–97S.
7. Russell, A. D. (1986) Mechanisms of resistance to antiseptics, disinfectants and preservatives. *Pharmacy International*, 7: 305–308.
8. Otter, J. A., et al. (2015) Surface-attached cells, biofilms and biocide susceptibility: Implications for hospital cleaning and disinfection. *Journal of Hospital Infection*, 89(1): 16–27.
9. Gram, L., Baggge-Ravn, D., Ng, Y.Y., Gymoese, P. and Vogel, B.F. (2007) Influence of food soiling matrix on cleaning and disinfection efficiency on surface attached Listeria monocytogenes. *Food Control*, 18: 1165–1171.
10. Sandle, T. (2016) The importance of detergent selection. *The Clinical Services Journal*, 15(8): 72–74.
11. Sandle, T. (2010) Choosing disinfectants. *Cleanroom Technology*, 18(8): 11–13.
12. McDonnell, G. and Russell, A. (1999) Antiseptics and disinfectants: Activity, action and resistance. *Clinical Microbiology Reviews*, January: 147–179.
13. Angelillo, I. F., Bianco, A., Nobile, C.G.A., and Pavia, M. (1998) Evaluation of the efficacy of glutaraldehyde and peroxygen for disinfection of dental instruments. *Letters in Applied Microbiology*, 27: 292–296.
14. Ernst, C. et al. (2006) Efficacy of amphoteric surfactant – and peracetic acid–based disinfectants on spores of *bacillus cereus in vitro* and on food premises of the German armed forces. *Journal of Food Protection*, 69(7): 1605–1610.
15. Antony, M. J. and Jayakannan, M. (2007) Amphiphilic azobenzenesulfonic acid anionic surfactant for water-soluble, ordered, and luminescent polypyrrole nanospheres. *Journal of Physical Chemistry B*, 111(44): 12772–12780.
16. Wilson, L. A., Sawant, A. D., and Ahearn, D. G. (1991) Comparative efficacies of soft contact lens disinfectant solutions against microbial films in lens cases. *Archives of Ophthalmology*, 109(8): 1155–1157.
17. Bergan, T. and Lystad, A. (1972): Evaluation of disinfectant inactivators. *Acta Pathalogica Microbiologica Scandinavica Section B*, 80: 507–510.
18. Vijayakumar, R., Kannan, V.V., Sandle, T., and Manoharan, C. (2012) *In vitro* antifungal efficacy of biguanides and quaternary ammonium compounds against cleanroom fungal isolates. *PDA Journal of Pharmaceutical Science and Technology*, 66(3): 236–242.
19. Gundheim, G., Langsrud, S., Heir, E., and Holck, A. L. (1998) Bacterial resistance to disinfectants containing quaternary ammonium compounds. *International Biodeterioration & Biodegradation*, 41(3–4): 235–239.
20. Sagripanti, J. L. and Bonifacino, A. (1996) Comparative sporicidal effect of liquid chemical germicides on three medical devices contaminated with spores of *Bacillus subtilis*. *American Journal of Infection Control*, 24: 364–371.

21. Sagripanti, J. L. and Bonifacino, A. (1996) Comparative sporicidal effects of liquid chemical agents. *Applied and Environmental Microbiology*, 62: 545–551.
22. Lensing, H. H. and Oei, H. L. (1985) Investigations on the sporicidal and fungicidal activity of disinfectants. Zentralblatt fur Bakteriologie, Mikrobiologie und Hygiene – 1 – Abt – *Originale B, Hygiene*, 181: 487–495.
23. Sandle, T. (2012) A new wave of sporicidal disinfectants. *Clean Air and Containment Review*, Issue 10: 10–13.
24. Larson, E. (1988) A causal link between handwashing and risk of infection? Examination of the evidence. *Control Hospital Epidemiology*, 9: 28–36.
25. Walsh, C. (2000). Molecular mechanisms that confer antibacterial drug resistance, *Nature*, 406: 775–781.
26. Abdallah, M., et al. (2015) Impact of growth temperature and surface type on the resistance of Pseudomonas aeruginosa and Staphylococcus aureus biofilms to disinfectants. *International Journal of Food Microbiology*, 214: 38–47.
27. Holah, J. T. (2003) Cleaning and disinfection. In Lelieveld, H. L. M., Mostert, M.A., Holah, J., and White, B. (Eds.) *Hygiene in Food Processing*, Woodhead Publishing Limited: Cambridge, UK, pp 235–278.
28. Sandle, T. (2015) Safe use of disinfectants and detergents in cleanrooms. *Innovation into Success* (quarterly journal of UKSPA), Issue 38: 81–84.
29. Sandle, T. (2014) Selection and use of cleaning and disinfection agents in pharmaceutical manufacturing. In Handlon, G. and Sandle, T. (Eds.) *Industrial Pharmaceutical Microbiology: Standards & Controls*, Euromed Communications: Passfield, UK, pp 9.1–9.32.
30. Panousi, M. N., Williams, G.J., Girdlestone, S., Hiom, S., and Maillard, J.Y. (2009) Evaluation of alcohol wipes used during aseptic manufacturing. *Letters in Allied Microbiology*, 48: 648–651.
31. Sutton, S. V. W. (2008) Disinfectant rotation in a cleaning/disinfection program for cleanrooms and controlled environments. In Manivannan, G. (Ed.) *Disinfection and Decontamination: Principles, Applications and Related Issues*, CRC Press, pp 165–174.
32. Denyer, S. P. and Stewart G. S. A. B. (1998) Mechanisms of action of disinfectants, *International Biodeterioration and Biodegradation*, 41: 261–268.
33. Russell, A. D. (1995) Mechanisms of bacterial resistance to biocides. *International Biodeterioration & Biodegradation*, 36(3–4): 247–265.
34. Bessems, E. (1998) The effect of practical conditions on the efficacy of disinfectants. *International Biodeterioration and Biodegradation*, 41: 177–183.
35. Baird, R. (1981) Cleaning and disinfection in the hospital pharmacy in Collins et al disinfectants, their use and evaluation of effectiveness. *Society Applied Bacteriology*, TS16: 154.
36. Sandle, T. (2012) Application of disinfectants and detergents in the pharmaceutical sector. In Sandle, T. (Ed.) *The CDC Handbook: A Guide to Cleaning and Disinfecting Cleanrooms*, Grosvenor House Publishing: Surrey, UK, pp 168–197.
37. Rotter, M. (1977) Alkohole fur eine Standarddes-infektionsmethode in der Wertbestimmung von Verfahren fur die HygienischeHandedesinfektion. *Zbl.Bakt. Hyg.*, B 164: 428–438.
38. Pharmaceutical Inspection and Co-operation Scheme. PIC/S PI 007-6 – Recommendation on the Validation of Aseptic Processes. Geneva, Switzerland, 2011.
39. US Food and Drug Administration Guidance for Industry – Sterile Drug Products Produced by Aseptic Processing, Current Good Manufacturing Practice. Bethesda, MD, USA, 2004.
40. Bloomfield, S. F. and Looney, E. (1992) Evaluation of the repeatability and reproducibility of European suspension test methods for antimicrobial activity of disinfectants and antiseptics. *Journal of Applied Bacteriology*, 73: 87–93.

41. Vina, P., Rubio, S. and Sandle, T. (2011) Selection and validation of disinfectants. In Saghee, M. R., Sandle, T., and Tidswell, E. C. (Eds.) *Microbiology and Sterility Assurance in Pharmaceuticals and Medical Devices*, Business Horizons: New Delhi, pp 219–236.

42. ASTM International, E2614-15: Standard Guide for Evaluation of Cleanroom Disinfectants. West Conshohocken, PA, USA, 2015.

43. United States Pharmacopeia. Chapter USP <1072> Antiseptics and Disinfectants. United States Pharmacopeia, Edition, 39: 1118–1123.

44. Tomasino, S. F. and Hamilton, M. A. (2006) Modification to the AOAC sporicidal activity of disinfectants test (Method 966.04): Collaborative study. *Journal of AOAC International*, 89: 1373–1397.

45. Sutton, S. V. W., Proud, D., Rachiu, S., and Brannan, S. K. (2002) Validation of microbial recovery from disinfectants. *PDA Journal of Pharmaceutical Science and Technology*, 56(5): 255–266.

46. Miyano, N., Oie, S., and Kamiya, K. (2003) Efficacy of disinfectants and hot water against biofilm cells of *burkholderia cepacian*. *Biological and Pharmaceutical Bulletin*, 26(5): 671–674.

47. Lloyd-Evans, N., Springthorpe, V. S., and Sattar, S. A. (1986) Chemical disinfection of human rotavirus-contaminated inanimate surfaces Journal of Hygiene, 97: 163–173.

48. Sandle, T. (2012) Validation of disinfectants. In Sandle, T. (Ed.) *The CDC Handbook: A Guide to Cleaning and Disinfecting Cleanrooms*, Grosvenor House Publishing: Surrey, UK, pp 241–261.

49. Sandle, T. (2012) Ensuring contamination control: The validation of disinfectants. *European Medical Hygiene*, November 2012: 33–39.

50. Vijayakumar, R., et al. (2016) Determination of minimum inhibitory concentrations of common biocides to multidrug-resistant gram-negative bacteria. *Applied Medical Research*, 2(3): 56–62.

51. Akhmaltdinova, L. L., Azizov, I., Sandle, T., Gyurka, A.G., and Chessca, A. (2016) Use of flow cytometry for the evaluation of disinfectant effectiveness. *Archives of the Balkan Medical Union*, 51(2): 213–215.

52. Sandle, T. (2011) A review of cleanroom microflora: Types, trends, and patterns. *PDA Journal of Pharmaceutical Science and Technology*, 65(4): 392–403.

53. Tidswell, E. C. (2005) Bacterial adhesion: considerations within a risk-based approach to cleaning validation. *PDA Journal of Pharmaceutical Science and Technology*, 59(1): 10–32.

3 Disinfecting Agents
The Art of Disinfection

Arthur Vellutato, Jr.

CONTENTS

3.1   INTRODUCTION

The art of disinfection has been successfully accomplished since the early 1800s in a multitude of capacities. Disinfectants, or rather, antimicrobial agents have long been in our world. They are found naturally in our environment and are created synthetically by humans. They range from mild, safely ingestible chemistries to toxic and corrosive agents that would most certainly produce a lethal effect in humans. But as with many things in the modern world, confusion surrounding where, when, and how antimicrobial agents are employed is commonplace. Complexities such as effectiveness, toxicity, corrosion, labeling, residuals, overuse, vapors, shipment, and suitability all cause confusion. Of more concern is the "lack of knowledge" factor that is further complicated by our continuation of past practices instead of current best science, our belief that what is said or required by regulatory agencies is correct, and our overall lack of complete understanding of the limitations of such antimicrobial agents. Every day such agents are most certainly inappropriately used, with a consequences that are detrimental to humans, our final product, our facilities, and the ecosystem at large.

There are a great number of registered drug products, over the counter drug products, soaps, creams, gels, foams, cleaners, fabrics, building materials, plants, animal extractants, and even paints with antimicrobial claims. And more and more products are being added to the list claiming antimicrobial properties. In one sense, this progress is good but it is also worrying that most people may never read the label on such products. We tend to read the big words: the product name or subtitle claim. We just pour some in a bucket with a "glug, glug" theory of measure and assume more is better. Directions for correct dilutions and solution and container disposal are ignored. This lack of detail leads us to misuse.

As an example, the most notable misinterpreted claim is a product that "kills 99% of household germs". Most assume that means that 99% of the organisms in the world are destroyed by the agent. But they are not. This statement means that 99% of the organisms that were tested, and at the population which they were tested were proven to be destroyed by the agent to a level of 99%. This leaves 1% of each organism tested still alive.

The pharmaceutical, biotechnology, healthcare, and lab animal world are no different than the consumer world in this venue. We scramble to find the most efficacious chemical but ignore the real art of disinfection that would most certainly assure success. We happily follow past practices and ignore any past imperfection and do not consider potential future practices. As we cling tightly to the way it was always done we potentially overuse our antimicrobial agents in both active ingredients and frequency. We fill our cleanrooms with residues that are difficult to completely remove. And, we place our personnel using such products in uncomfortable and possibly adverse health situations. And we corrode our expensive equipment and surfaces due to over use and lack of true cleaning. Often we choose the quick answer and discard the reliable more involved method as we rush to complete our task to either get our operations back in motion or to meet the all-important CAPA (corrective and preventative actions) deadline. And in doing so, we sacrifice science for completion.

3.2   DISINFECTION PROCESS AT A GLANCE

Disinfection is a general term that is used to describe the destruction of a micro-organism. But the term is also used in a singular, noun format of disinfectant to describe a classification of agents that prove efficacy of certain vegetative cells. The dually used term causes some confusion but this connotation has been used since the beginning of antimicrobial agents and will most likely never be changed. The destruction of a cell on a hard surface or in liquid is based on the saturation and penetration of the cell wall or an organism with an efficacious chemical agent, for a specific contact time. Concern is vested in the potential soil load on the surface or the liquid to be disinfected that may either compromise the contact of the chemical agent to the organism or may soak up the actives in the chemical agent preventing it from not contacting the cell. Most agents work on the theory of cytoplasmic disruption whereby the actives penetrate the cell and explode the nucleus. The penetration is dependent upon surface contact of the chemical agent to the exterior of the cell and a contact or wetted time sufficient to allow this penetration or saturation to occur.

Disinfection is effective in many places and in other places virtually impossible. On hard surfaces in a clean room disinfection is normally successful but at different levels based on the surface type. A hard surface like stainless steel provides very little surface irregularity, however a more porous surface like epoxy, plastic, vinyl, Mipolam®, Kidex®, ceramic, and plexiglass presents a more difficult challenge. Microorganisms can vest themselves into pores inherent in the surface and this contact with the disinfectant on a sufficient surface area also becomes more of a challenge. At the same time dirtied surfaces may block the chemical agent from reaching the surface of an organism as the organism may be vested in a pore or imperfection of the surface and surrounded by a soil load.

In the venue of disinfection, surfaces are categorized in several types. Metals are the easiest surfaces to disinfect. Glass and plexiglass can have pores and can present minimum problems. Epoxy, Terrazo®, Mipolam®, Kidex®, vinyl, and like surfaces present further problems as pores and imperfections are more prevalent in the makeup of the surface. These surfaces trap more particulate, foreign matter and residuals and can further complicate disinfection. Ceramic, tile, grout, polymers, sealers, and many plastics create an even more difficult challenge as they have further imperfection and pore issues that act as previously described to block contact of the agent or vest contaminants in such imperfections. Cloth, foam, uncoated or poorly coated dry wall, concrete, cinderblock, paper, and other cellulose and noncellulose product that incorporates the ability to soak up water or contamination have an enormous potential to vest organisms that may never be reached by chemical agents. These surfaces present the greatest challenge and in some instances, especially with mold infestation. If contaminated with mold such surfaces may never be disinfected as the mold reaches deep into the pores and the surface may become virtually impossible disinfect. In this situation, removal of the surfaces or structures may be the only option.

Disinfection of air is virtually impossible. Many think that vapors or spray into the air is effective, but it is not. The inability of the organism to become saturated for any length of time suitable for destruction of the cell simply cannot occur. And thus, contact time or dry time is too short. Disinfection of air is normally engineered from an air filtration process. However, filtration cannot assist when contamination is allowed to be continuously introduced to the clean room. As an example, imagine you are an organism on a particle that came in through a door from the outside. First you have to avoid all the obstacles in the clean room. Next, you have to navigate your way through the currents inherent and created in the clean room so you can make your way to the return vent. But air keeps pushing you down and people keep blowing you left and right. Now, the entire time you are floating you have one thing in mind: finding food, water, and surviving. You find food in particulates and other organisms, and the search for food is your main direction to sustain life. So most likely you will land on a surface as the potential for available food is greater. However, if you do not you next have to avoid the covering of the return vent and be taken on a road trip through the heating, ventilation, and air conditioning (HVAC) process to the filter in the ceiling where most likely you will be retained. As explained, the removal of airborne microorganisms is a difficult challenge. Gassing systems can assist but again, you have to create a toxic environment whereby the air is of a corrosive nature to the cell and due to this, over time, you will have either a chemical disruption on the wall of the cell or deplete the cell of oxygen. Processes like vaporized hydrogen peroxide (VHP) in this venue is not toxic enough and if you were to be able to create such a toxic environment you would most certainly simultaneously create an extremely toxic environment for humans. Such processes are effective for surface disinfection provided that shadowing and other criteria are met completely. And the surface is never cleaned by fogging or gassing. If one seeks to destroy an organism that can survive without oxygen, called an aerotolerant organism, or the more used slang term of "anaerobic organism", depletion of oxygen from the clean room is necessary to assure its demise. This is seen in processes with nitrogen blankets as a means of removal of oxygen from the area. Again, a practice that could not be vested in the entire facility but only a localized area and in the end also does not clean the surface. The only truly assured methodology to destroy or rather prevent an airborne organism is control.

While we focus in this chapter on antimicrobial agents it is extremely important to realize that the agent alone cannot assure an acceptable environment. A wholistic approach therefore needs to be invoked to assure we can attain what we desire— acceptable environmental conditions to meet product and regulatory requirements. This means you are going to have to go further than spreading some antimicrobial agents onto the surface. In fact, the firm that controls more and disinfects less always wins the battle. The firm that decides to have minimal control and disinfects more to combat the invasion of contamination seems to always have excursions that riddle operations with expensive investigations, placing band aids on unsound practices and routine regulatory comments. Truly, the wholistic approach is the desired means to the end.

3.3 TERMINOLOGY—SANITIZERS, DISINFECTANTS, SPORICIDES, AND STERILANTS

The varying terminology surrounding disinfection and disinfectants worldwide is one of the most confusing aspects in the scope of the subject matter. So much confusion is created initially by governmental agencies, industry, labeling, shipping regulations, safety data sheets (SDS), and past beliefs. One may ask why is this so? The answer is very simple. Each country has its own set of rules for how disinfectants will be registered, tested, and labeled. To add to this confusion, past beliefs coupled with varying regulatory comments contradict each other and create terminology confusion. Later in this chapter these regulatory discrepancies between agencies will be discussed in detail.

For the good manufacturing practice (GMP) professional, only four terminologies are required to be understood. These are: Sanitizer, Disinfectant, Sporicidal Product and Sporicide/Cold Sterilant. All have different meanings and characteristics, however, the slang terminology used for all of these terms is "disinfectant". Definitions for each are presented below.

3.3.1 SANITIZER

Sanitizer is a compound that will reduce the number of bacteria to a safe level. Determined by the US Environmental Protection Agency (EPA) as *Escherlchia coli* and *Salmonella typhi*, or *Staphylococcus aureus* for food product contact surfaces. For example: 70% IPA or EtOH.

3.3.2 DISINFECTANT

Disinfectant is a chemical or physical agent that destroys or removes vegetative forms of harmful microorganisms. Determined by the US EPA as 10^6 reduction of *Salmonella cholerasuis, Staphylococcus aureus*, and *Pseudomonas aeruginosa* on stainless penicylinders with the presence of a soil load. For example: phenol or quats.

3.3.3 SPECIFIC SPORICIDAL PRODUCT

Specific sporicidal product is a compound that when tested destroys a particular organism at an acceptable level as defined by registering bodies. An example of this would be "Sporicidal Against *Clostridium difficile* (*C. Diff)*". Determined by the EPA as the 10^6 reduction of *Clostridium difficile* or the organism claimed is required on penicylinders with the presence of a soil load. For example: lower level peroxides, bleaches and PA H_2O_2.

3.3.4 SPORICIDE/COLD STERILANT

Sporicide/cold sterilant a compound that destroys all vegetative microorganism and bacterial and fungal spores. Determined by the EPA as the 10^6 reduction of *Bacillus subtilis* and *Clostridium sporogenes* on stainless penicylinders with the presence of a soil load. For example: bleach or PA H_2O_2

So what's the real difference between these compounds, chemicals, or physical agents? A sanitizer is the weakest of the claims. In this classification are alcohols that can be used during manufacturing. Every other class, compound, or agent should not be used during manufacturing due to the possibility of residuals contaminating final product, overspray of possibly toxic agents that may enter product, harmful and toxic vapors, and most importantly the contamination of gloves with possibly toxic or harmful agents that can cause problems during aseptic manipulations or handling of aseptic connections.

A disinfectant, by its true definition, is a chemical that destroys vegetative cells and has little effect on spores, if any. And such an agent is used routinely because the routine use of the specific sporicide or the sporicide/cold sterilant can cause significant corrosion of surfaces when used at that frequency. The use of the specific sporicide or the sporicide/cold sterilant daily to address contamination noticed in environmental monitoring signals a control problem and not an infestation of spores that linger in the room. The specific sporicide should be considered a dangerously claimed product if the end-user is not paying attention as it is only valuable for the spore which is listed and not all spores. It does not have the broad efficacy performance required for the sporicide/cold sterilant. Many products like this claim a specific spore is killed such as *Clostridium difficile* (*C. Diff*) which in reality is very easy to destroy. The testing only needs to be done on carrier surfaces and not sutures like the sporicide/cold sterilant. End users should read the label to see what exactly the agent is capable of destroying prior to use. The assumption that it destroys all spores is incorrect. The sporicide/cold sterilant is the strongest label claim and to destroy *Bacillus subtilis* and *Clostridium sporogenes* it requires a minimum of 1.0×10^6 in a blood serum soil load. This claim requires surfaces and suture testing to be performed and is the strongest claim available.

3.4   CONTAMINATION CONTROL

Maintaining control of the environment is critical. It is the most important aspect surrounding a cleaning and disinfection program. We need to understand that control of the environment does not come from using a chemical agent that will destroy all microorganisms. Rather, control of the environment is the assurance level we establish to reduce or possibly eliminate the contamination from ever entering our controlled areas. Once a chemical agent has been applied to the surface and subsequently dries, its destructive capabilities to a microorganism are complete. Disinfection (or sporicidal) characteristics of a chemical agent require the organism to be wetted by the agent. While certain residues from chemical agents may have some remaining antimicrobial properties, the destructive capabilities of the residue are minimal. Control over what enters the controlled area now takes over. Control of the environment has nothing to do with disinfection. Disinfection is complete when control takes over. Manufacturing operations will not disinfect surfaces while production is occurring. Disinfection is done prior to manufacturing and the environment released to produce a product. Our success or failure in control is measured each time as environmental monitoring is conducted during our filling operations.

By addressing contamination prior to its entry will assure we will not have to contend with its presence. While disinfection of surfaces always takes the lead in structuring our procedures, control over the environment should remain one of our main focuses.

Criteria for reducing the bioburden that enters the controlled area requires us to evaluate the entry of personnel, components, water, tanks, carts, and even disinfectants to name a few. This is done to assure that we do not undermine our disinfection efforts by introducing high levels of contamination after disinfection is complete. We must assure each item's appropriateness in the room classification to which it enters. In Grade A/B aseptic operations, we need to careful evaluate each item as clean and sterile prior to entry. We need to assure the cleanliness, sterility and appropriate fit of garments for our personnel. In Grade C/D, while our concern is less we must assure that such environmental conditions do not adversely affect the Grade A/B area. In short, a room can be monitored as having very little if any bioburden at rest, however, in a static condition we can easily corrupt our efforts previously achieved through poor control.

3.5   CLEANING VERSUS DISINFECTION

Too often cleaning is confused with disinfection. They are not the same. Cleaning characterizes the removal of particulates, microbes, and possibly existent residues from surfaces. Cleaning requires a nondestructive mechanical action be applied that loosens and removes contaminants from the area. Procedurally, contaminates and residues are loosened and rinsed to the floor. Subsequently, the dirtied solution on the floor is collected and removed from the area (normally by a squeegee). By lessening the level of particulates, microbes, and residues on the surface, our disinfection efforts become simpler. First there are fewer organisms to destroy as most have been removed from the area. And secondly, as bioburden and residues are lower, the possible obstructions blocking the chemical agent from contacting the organism are minimized. In short, cleaning prepares the surface for disinfection.

Disinfection relates to the saturation and penetration of the cell wall of an organism by a chemical agent. It further requires that an organism remain wetted for a specified contact time with a chemical agent capable of killing the organism in question. Disinfection depends upon temperature, saturation and penetration of the cell wall, contact time, surface and bioburden of the surface, existent soil load, concentration of the chemical agent, and pH. Provided the appropriate chemical agent is utilized, the key to disinfection in the clean room is keeping the surface wetted for 5–10 minutes. This is difficult, as the movement of air via laminar flow tends to dry surfaces quicker.

As discussed, there is a significant difference between cleaning and disinfection. Cleaning tries to remove contamination from the surface while disinfection attempts to destroy what viable cells exist on the surface. We can use a toothbrush and mouthwash as real-life examples. If we were to discuss the options of not using a toothbrush anymore and only utilizing a daily mouthwash rinse with our dentist, he/she would inform us that we would soon have no teeth. Residues, particulates and microbials will build up on the surface of our teeth and they would eventually deteriorate. This scenario depicts what occurs too often in the pharmaceutical and biotechnology industry. We forget to brush and just try to kill anything that exists on the surface. Eventually our surfaces become residue laden and more difficult to disinfect and eventually deteriorate. Within our note to technical brilliance we sometimes forget simple common sense. And unfortunately, the phrase, "simple common sense" is not the title of any good manufacturing practice (GMP), Code of Federal Regulations (CFR), or guidance document.

The effect of the buildup of residues, particulates, and possibly microbials is also aided by the surface itself. Clean room surfaces are irregular in nature as depicted in the scanning electron microscope (SEM) photos within this chapter. Such surfaces trap residues and other contaminants and make the surface more difficult to disinfect. (See SEM photos of residues and surfaces throughout this chapter).

Sooner or later we have to clean. The frequency of cleaning can vary from a daily function to a monthly function. It is usual to clean surfaces either bi-weekly or on a monthly basis. Some may say, "But that's an additional cleaning operation we need to do". The correct response is "It needs to be done".

Within the healthcare setting and most commonly reported in the hospital setting, test reports have shown the effect that cleaning the surface has on the microbial levels in controlled areas. Many publications purport this concept. In the pharmaceutical and biotechnology setting, a test report conducted and published in 1989 by A. Vellutato, Sr. and A. Vellutato, Jr. of Veltek Associates, Inc. demonstrated the effect cleaning the surfaces has on the level of microbial contamination found on the surface. The study focused on the concept that cleaning alone would remove most of the existing microbial contamination. In the report, all surfaces were cleaned with a sodium lauryl sulfate detergent and mechanical cleaning action on a daily basis. Such cleaning was conducted in a Grade A/B, Grade A, ISO 5 area. Environmental monitoring was routinely conducted at air, surface, and personnel sampling locations. The manufacturing operations filled an average of 4,000 units of 500 ml bags of USP water-for-injection. Manufacturing operations ran for four hours per day and upon completion of manufacturing, the clean room was completely cleaned. The cleaning mechanism utilized a mop and two-bucket system, a sprayer, and a squeegee. The procedure for cleaning was to apply the sodium lauryl sulfate detergent (DECON-Clean®) to the surface utilizing a top to bottom approach. Upon completion of the mopping, the chemical was then sprayed on to the surface and all excess liquid on the surfaces pulled downward by squeegee to the floor. The remaining liquid was then collected on the floor and removed. The results for 30 days met industry limits for Grade A/B, Grade A, ISO 5. At 45 days, control was lost, results exceeded limits and a sporicidal agent was used once on day 45. The limits returned to acceptable levels for 31 days (day 76 of the study). The final conclusion was one to two uses of a sporicidal agent with the cleaning regime controlled the environment.

Cleaning is based on a few physical factors; 1) the surface to be cleaned, 2) the contamination vested on the surface, 3) the chemical used to clean the surface, 4) the effect of the chemical agent on the surface to be cleaned, 5) the level of surfactants in the chemical agent, and 6) the effect of the chemical on the contamination, moreover residue, that exists on the surface.

Knowledge of the type of surface to be cleaned is very important. And, it is important to understand the concept of surface irregularity, surface tension, and residue build up so that when antimicrobial effectiveness studies are performed one can account for these inconsistencies. As depicted in Figures 3.1–3.6, surface irregularity varies as composite materials change. The surface irregularity may compromise

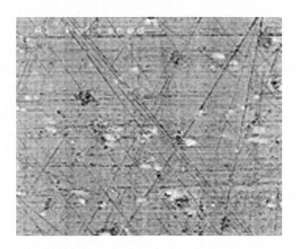

FIGURE 3.1 Aluminum Surface.

FIGURE 3.2 Stainless Steel Surface.

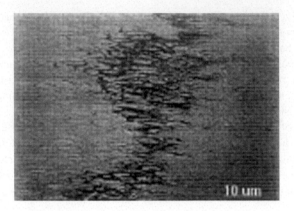

FIGURE 3.3   Epoxy Coated Surface.

cleaning and disinfection efforts for two basic reasons. First, cleaning becomes more difficult. And second, disinfection becomes harder as the chemical agent cannot contact all the surfaces for the required wetted time period (as obstructions may exist). Cleaning becomes more difficult as the surface's irregular nature may allow particulates, residues, and even microbial contamination to vest itself within the rutted or porous areas of the surface. These "nooks and crannies" are very hard to clean with most clean room apparatus designed for cleaning. Most clean room mops and wipes are flat and do not allow the penetration of the fibers or surfaces of the cleaning mechanism to reach into the crevices. The lack of such an abrasive cleaning action bypasses the opportunity to loosen and remove these contaminants. Most irregular surfaces are commonly so across the span of the material, so a multitude of contamination sources exist on the surface to be cleaned. Cleaning of an irregular surface

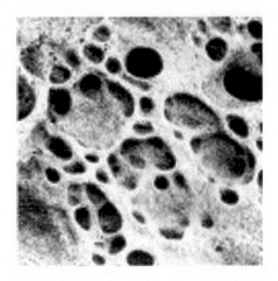

FIGURE 3.4   Clean Room Curtains #1.

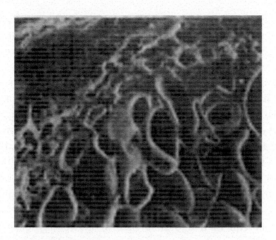

FIGURE 3.5   Clean Room Curtains #2.

requires one to use a cleaning device that can penetrate into the "nooks and crannies" and make contact with the existent contaminants and residues. As an example, we would not use a wiper or a pad to try to clean our teeth. We would use a toothbrush. Unfortunately, a clean room brush is not a commonly available item in the industry. Nor would requiring a controlled area to be cleaned with it be a reasonable request of production personnel. This is a subject that the cleaning apparatus manufacturers need to address more closely. The lack of available products forces the clean room professional to adapt a non-clean room product to address this specific need.

The second basic complication is that if particulates and residues exist in such "nooks and crannies", the possibility for a disinfecting agent to contact the surface within the "nooks and crannies" is improbable. Thus, we are disinfecting the surface of the particulates and residues and never disinfecting the actual surface. Without such assurance for cleaning and disinfecting the actual surface, the possibility for contamination to be vested underneath the particulate and residue may be probable.

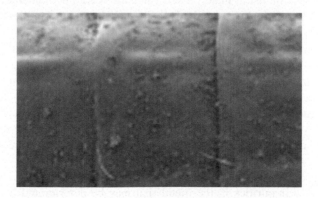

FIGURE 3.6   Vinyl Surface.

In the upcoming sections of this chapter we will discuss antimicrobial effectiveness testing. In these sections we will come to understand that during such validation testing we need to look to inoculate a surface with a known enumeration of microorganisms and soak such surfaces in a disinfecting agent for a predetermined time period. Upon completion of the soaking, we will then test the surface to account for the possibly remaining viable contamination. When we attempt to use such data in the field, we will find our testing skewed for two basic factors. First, our testing inoculates a variety of surfaces with a multitude of microorganisms. Some surfaces are more irregular than others. In our test, and after we have soaked the surfaces, we need to rinse clean the surfaces of any possible contamination to a filter which is then plated to a growth medium. However, we find the rinsing of the irregular surfaces more difficult as microorganisms may vest and cling within the irregular areas of the surface. This means the possibility to rinse free a microorganism from a smooth surface is easier than from an irregular surface. What we may learn from this testing is that it may seem that our disinfecting agent is more effective on the irregular or porous surface, but this is due to our inability to rinse free all of the existent microorganisms. The smooth surfaces are more easily rinsed and existent microorganisms removed and can grow in our growth medium. However, the microorganisms from the irregular or porous surface may have never been removed from the surface itself. This means they were never rinsed to the filter and plated for growth. Thus, we could conclude smooth surfaces are harder to disinfect than irregular or porous surfaces in our manufacturing and testing areas. The effectiveness report may show higher remaining colony forming units (CFUs) for the smooth surfaces than the irregular or porous surfaces. This assumption would be incorrect. In the manufacturing or testing areas the opposite occurs, and we find it more difficult to disinfect the irregular or porous surfaces. Understanding this concept is critical to successful disinfection. We will have the same trouble, if not a more complicated problem, in disinfecting and rinsing the microorganisms from the irregular or porous surfaces in our manufacturing and testing areas. And due to this, we may leave viable contamination on such surfaces. Care needs to be taken when disinfecting irregular or porous surfaces, as they are harder to clean and disinfect than smoother surfaces.

In general, clean room material grades can be separated into six basic categories. While a more specific list of material sub-categories could be rendered, for our discussion and understanding we can divide them into: aluminum, stainless steel, epoxy coated finishes, plastics, vinyl, and glass.

In Figure 3.1, we see an aluminum surface. This surface is a metal grade that is soft and easily scratches and is deteriorated by chlorine solutions, glutaraldehyde and peroxide, and peracetic acid and hydrogen peroxide solutions (from a list of basic disinfecting agents). While aluminum is a commonly used metal, deterioration of the surface from chemical exposure normally shows as a turquoise bluish gray bubbling on the metal. Aluminum is also easily stained or discolored from the residues from by phenol, quaternary ammonium, and iodine to name a few. However, of most clean room surfaces, aluminum is normally easy to clean and disinfect.

In Figure 3.2, we see a 316 L stainless steel surface. This surface is very smooth and contains few impurities in the metal that may be deteriorated by a disinfecting agent. Most impurities in the metal grade are that of the carbon family and are deteriorated by chlorine solutions, glutaraldehyde and peroxide, and peracetic acid and hydrogen peroxide solutions (from a list of basic disinfecting agents). Stainless comes in grade based on the level of impurities in the metal. Normally deterioration of the surface is in the form of a rusting that pits the surface or surface rust. Rusting of the stainless itself is from chemicals or water oxidizing and/or reacting with impurities in the metal. Surface rust is the rusting of airborne heavy metals that deposit atop the surface. Within the clean room operation, many metal grades exist from of 302 to 402 stainless. Many in the industry demand the use of 316 L stainless, however this metal grade cannot be used for every component due to its brittle nature. Some perfect examples of this would be a spring or a solenoid mechanism. Utilizing a metal too hard will cause the spring or moving part to routinely break as friction of movement on the metal will cause stress and fracture. Stainless is also easily stained or discolored from the residues from by phenol, quaternary ammonium, and iodine to name a few. However, among clean room surfaces, stainless steel is normally one of the easiest surfaces to clean and disinfect.

In Figure 3.3, we see an epoxy coated surface. Epoxy type surfaces are very numerous in types and materials. They are a coating that is applied in a liquid form and then hardens. This is where disinfection becomes complicated. Its irregular surface appearance makes epoxy challenging for the disinfection professional. Most clean room walls and floors are made of an epoxy material or similar material so understanding cleaning and disinfection of this surface is critical. Common build up of particulates and moreover residues in the crevices complicate cleaning and disinfection. Problematic situations can arise in the crevices of the surfaces as air pockets can form and, once disinfection is complete, be broken and possibly release existent contamination to the environment. The most difficult task with the epoxy coated surface is to clean the contaminants from the surface so that the disinfectant can be applied and have the ability to address the surface itself. Normally epoxy coated surfaces are deteriorated by chlorine solutions, peroxide, isopropyl alcohol, ethanol, and peracetic acid and hydrogen peroxide solutions (from a list of basic disinfecting agents). The normal deterioration occurs in the form of over drying and cracking of the material finish. The material becomes powder-like and orange to blue in color (dependent upon the material). Epoxy coated surfaces need routine replacement or refinishing and as such remain continuously on a preventative maintenance schedule. The epoxy coated finish is also easily stained or discolored from the residues from phenol, quaternary ammonium, and iodine to name a few.

The next basic clean room surface type is a collage or porous material such as plastic, vinyl, plexiglass, delron, and other similar type products. In Figure 3.4, 3.5 and 3.6 we can see what these surfaces may look like when magnified through an SEM microscope. Characteristically they have pore openings that are rather deep. Cleaning and disinfection are very difficult with these materials. Normally these types of surfaces need to be replaced over time. These materials average about two to three years before requiring replacement. Replacement is costly but required and should be viewed as a cost of doing business. Normally porous surfaces are deteriorated by chlorine solutions, peroxide, isopropyl alcohol, ethanol, and peracetic acid and hydrogen peroxide solutions (from a list of basic disinfecting agents). The normal deterioration occurs in the form of over drying and cracking of the material itself. A yellowing or changing of color to an orange or brown are common symptoms of the drying process. The porous material is very easily stained or discolored from the residues from by phenol, quaternary ammonium, and iodine to name a few, and such residues and/or stains only increase the deterioration process. Most notably these materials are use as curtains that separate process control areas. Items such as plastic curtains are one of the most widely used materials in the clean room environment. Cleaning of these surfaces is normally done frequently if not daily as they represent the second closest non-product contact surface next to the filling line itself. This over cleaning shortens the life of the material.

The last category is glass. Glass is a relatively smooth surface with the characteristic of not deteriorating. Glass is very difficult to clean but remains a constant example of how difficult all surfaces are to clean. The reason glass seems harder to clean is one can see through it. All other materials discussed to this point are not clear. If such materials were clear, as is glass, the cleanliness of these surfaces would look horrifically dirtied in comparison to glass. Glass is very easily dirtied. It is a very difficult material to keep clean. However, this surface is used more and more each day in clean room operations as it allows viewing of the operation by supervisors and visitors. In general, glass does not stain easily from disinfectants or sporicides. However, residues build up and it is discolored from the residues of phenol, quaternary ammonium, and iodine to name a few.

We have seen from this section the importance of cleaning. In Figures 3.7–3.10 we can see what these culprit residuals look like through SEM photos. Simply, the

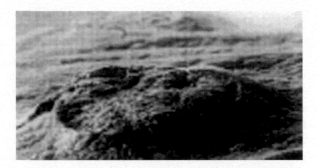

FIGURE 3.7   Phenolic Residue.

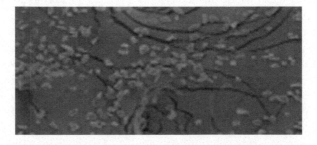

FIGURE 3.8   Sodium Chloride Residue.

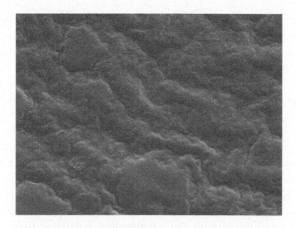

FIGURE 3.9   Quaternary Ammonium Residue.

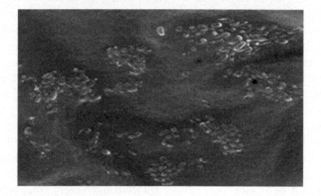

FIGURE 3.10   Peracetic Acid and H_2O_2 Residue.

effect of cleaning surfaces assures the best possible opportunity to disinfect the surface as the microbial levels and the possibly existent residues and particulates will be lower. Later in this chapter we will discuss the mechanisms to clean such surfaces. However, first we must understand the chemical agents that cause the main problem associated with a dirtied surface, the residue.

3.6   WORLDWIDE REGULATORY REQUIREMENTS FOR AGENTS AND GOOD MANUFACTURING PRACTICE (GMP)

As a subject, worldwide regulatory requirements could run to several books. Prior to the year 2002, the main worldwide registering bodies were the United States Environmental Protection Agency (EPA), the Australian Therapeutics Goods Administration (TGA), the Canadian Health Canada, the Chinese Ministry of Health (MOH) and several registering bodies that were country specific throughout Europe prior to the creation of the Biocidal Products Directive 98/8/EC (BPD). However, in recent years this list and the requirements for such registration throughout the world has exploded to a point where nearly every country seems to now have an authority for the registration of antimicrobial agents. While this controls chemical and process antimicrobials it also increases costs dramatically, lengthens approval times, institutes varying types of labeling, and most importantly tries to marry one requirement from one country to another which the world sees as virtually impossible.

Some of the most confusing scenarios in worldwide regulatory registration are labeling, varying claim requirements, and varying test procedures. Let us first discuss labeling. Well that is simple. Incorrect thinking would be to create the label and make it available in many languages and this should work for the world. Unfortunately, it is not that simple. Each country has a layout they desire. Most agree with the four-panel theory that places required labeling aspects into four distinct panels that each take up a side of the container. They are left, right, front, and back. While four panels are available, in some instances this does not provide enough space. Thus, putting secondary labeling material inside the label in a peel and reveal label format is normally acceptable where the container is too small or the text required is lengthy. The inconsistent part of labeling worldwide is that each country requires differing information on each panel. While the name of the brand, the subtitle claim, and the ingredients are standard on the front label, some desire first aid on the front panel and some on the side right or back panel. The remainder of the required label text is often different in each country. Label warnings like directions for use, precautionary statements, storage/disposal, general information, and efficacy performance are all located in varying sections on the label in every country. Unfortunately, there is not one approved standardized format for labels that can serve the world. This causes confusion for the end-user and moreover management who will write internal standard operating procedures (SOPs) and safety documents. A firm with multi-locations throughout the world will have to create separate documentation for each country even though they may be using the same product at each location as the pertinent locations for vital information is different in each country. Two other problems are the requirements for each country referencing the claim made on a product and the varying test procedures required to be used to make each claim for a product. And moreover, the main confusion is that the testing and approved label claims for efficacy performance really do not serve pharmaceutical, biotechnology, lab animal, or the compounding pharmacy industries. There are many standard tests that are employed by each country that include but are not limited to AOAC (Association of Official Analytical Chemists), Annex IIB and VI of the BPDEU or EN Testing (EU Biocidal Directive), and many ASTM test protocols (per country/product/claim). A firm registering an antimicrobial agent will have to register the product in virtually every country in the world and know that the hundreds of thousands of dollar spent, the time and effort incurred, and the final product information will not meet the requirements of a GMP facility. And as such, GMP operations will have to reconduct antimicrobial effectiveness testing accordingly to meet governmental regulations for drug products.

3.7 ANTIMICROBIAL EFFECTIVENESS

Determining what chemical agents will destroy a known level of one's environmental isolates or ATCC cultures is the next step. Prior to conducting either a Time Contact Kill Study (Tube Dilution), or a Time Contact Kill Study (On User Surfaces) or an AOAC Protocol Study, one needs to review the available disinfecting agents and determine which is initially appropriate for their operations. Upon choosing one or two disinfecting agents and a sporicide, one can continue with the antimicrobial effectiveness studies.

Validating one's sanitizing, disinfecting, and sporicidal agents requires them to delineate the organisms to be tested. One could use a list of ATCC cultures; however, utilization of one's environmental isolates nets a more exacting test for each unique manufacturing operation. Testing ATCC cultures such as *Bacillus subtilis*, *Aspergillus niger*, *Pseudomonas aeruginosa*, *Staphylococcus aureus*, *Candida albicans* and *Escherichia coli* is acceptable, however not as exacting as testing a plane of one's known environmental isolates. The use of one's environmental isolates in a preferred methodology by most regulatory agencies.

Antimicrobial effectiveness studies need to be based on realistic bioburdens that may be noticed in the controlled areas. It is usual is to test an enumeration greater than or equal to 1.0×10^4 CFUs. Our goal is to prove a three-log reduction. However, some guidelines like the British Standard BS EN 13697:2001 calls for a four-log reduction as proof.

In determining which test to conduct, one needs to review how one will address an organism in the clean room. As the organism will be on the surface, a time contact kill study that confirms the destruction of a known enumeration of cells on an end-user's surface is more depictive than a time contact kill study done in a tube dilution (in suspension). The reasoning for this is organisms dried on a surface better depict the situation of disinfecting an organism in the clean room. The available surface area of the organism that can be contacted by the disinfectant that rests on the surface is 270°. The available surface area of the organism that can be contacted by the disinfectant in the tube dilution study is 360°. Obviously, the surface test presents a more realistic scenario. AOAC protocol testing is required by the EPA to register a claim for a disinfecting agent. It utilizes 60 carriers (a ceramic penicylinder) and requires a high enumeration value of equal to or greater than 1.0×10^6. Protocols use either AOAC use-dilution or AOAC sporicidal tests procedures. While this is the method used for registration, it may be too involved and expensive for pharmaceutical and biotechnology firms to utilize as a method for testing antimicrobial effectiveness.

The EPA supports the use carrier methods for the evaluation of a disinfectant product's efficacy. This test requires the microorganism is to be dried on a nonporous carrier. The rationales behind the choice of a carrier method are the beliefs that (1) microorganisms that are dried are more difficult to chemically inactivate than those microorganisms in suspension, and (2) that in the health care setting microorganisms are more often found in the dried state than in suspension.

Within the framework of antimicrobial effectiveness testing, we also need to incorporate realistic contact times to depict representative dry times of the disinfectant on clean room surfaces. Due to the significant movement of air from laminar flow in the clean room, normal dry time is five minutes at best. While our floors may remain wetted longer (possibly up to ten minutes), the vertical surfaces will dry faster (three to five minutes). Thus, antimicrobial effectiveness testing should incorporate a worst-case scenario and utilize a three to five minutes dry time. An exception to this rule would be sanitizing agents such as isopropyl alcohol, ethyl alcohol or AAA ethanol at a concentration of 70%. These products dry faster nearing one to two minutes and testing should be altered as such. In recent years, many firms have begun to test three time frames to prove the disinfectant's activity over varying time periods. This author supports this practice and would suggest the time period of three, five and ten minutes be tested consecutively. Normally in three minutes the disinfectant shows average activity, in five minutes good activity, and in ten minutes excellent activity. Testing of a variety of times assures one has data in the file to support a complete range of dry times (contact times) that may be noticed in their manufacturing or testing operations. Upon completion, this testing will provide the justification for utilizing the chemical agents to destroy the known and possibly existent contamination in the facility. As time progresses, we need to continually update our profile of organisms versus our chemical agents.

While the type of test, the enumeration level of microorganisms, and the contact time are some of the most critical factors to assess, other critical factors also need to be determined. One of these is expiration of the disinfectant. Expiration for effectiveness can be determined by incorporating a simple variable in our test called aging of the disinfecting agent. Simply done, one would open a bottle of disinfectant and age it for the time period that they plan to use it, say 30-days (concentrate and ready-to-use). A ready-to-use solution is tested at the 30-day period. For a concentrate, the aged concentrate solution is diluted to the prescribed use-dilution. The use-dilution is then aged for the time period that it will be used (for example seven days). At the expiration of the use-dilution it is then tested for antimicrobial effectiveness. This system of expiration proves that a solution in use for "X" time period can destroy an acceptable level of microorganisms that we have determined to be present in our operations.

Expiration dating of disinfectant effectiveness can also be tested by conducting an antimicrobial effectiveness test on a newly open bottle of disinfectant (ready-to-use or concentrate to use-dilution) and then subsequently aging the solution for the expiry period and testing the active ingredients. The correlation between the active ingredients at time of opening and their satisfactory stability at end of expiry provides the needed data to support the use of the agent for the time period. However, in this test, there must be the understanding and explanation of the relationship between the tested solution and the expiry active data that followed.

In performing antimicrobial effectives testing some other factors come to the foreground that warrant attention. The first is soil load. Normally clean room operations do not have a soil load present and the most soil that exists would be that of disinfectant residues. In the case of an existing soil load, one should conduct their testing in a similar situation. Commonly used as a soil load or an increase level of protein (a fetal bovine serum) at 5% v/v is added to the organism challenge to test the ability of the disinfectant or sporicide under the circumstances of a soil load (dirtied) condition.

Another factor that may surface is hardness and temperature of water. Required by all registrants of disinfecting agents must state in their labeling their ability or inability to achieve antimicrobial effectiveness in the presence of hard water (400 p.p.m. as $CaCO_3$). At the same time the temperature of the solution may vary in its effect against microorganisms as elevated temperatures tend to increase the ability of the chemical agent's performance.

While disinfectant validations are expensive and time consuming they are foremost in most regulatory agency's minds. And thus, are required to assure the effectiveness of a cleaning and disinfection system that will prove an acceptable environment during the manufacture of product.

3.8 ASSAY OF DISINFECTING AGENTS

Analytical validation of our disinfecting agents' tests that the required percentage of the chemical agent is present to assure antimicrobial effectiveness. If the appropriate use instructions are followed, a ready-to-use product or a formulation from concentrate is normally easy to prove as having a sufficient amount of the active ingredients to reconfirm the required percentage that was validated in our antimicrobial effectiveness studies. Upon the use of this product past the first use is where we start to see the possibility that the percentage of the active ingredients may begin to slowly become too low to warrant continued use. Varying products have varying in-use time periods. Time periods range from seven to 30 days. This scenario needs to be validated for each chemical agent and each container type. As an example of the same chemical having varied in-use time periods, an iso-propyl alcohol solution in an aerosol for can be used for a longer time period than a trigger spray bottle. The reasoning for this difference is the aerosol container is sealed in a pressure vessel. The reduction in percentage of the active ingredient due to evaporation or the question of sterility over time is not founded in this container type. On the other hand, the trigger spray container may slowly aspirate room air to the master reservoir that may compromise the level of active ingredient and the sterility of the container over time. The basic validation question is what time frame we can prove the chemical's active percentage and sterility to be valid for, once opened.

3.9 STERILITY OF DISINFECTING AGENTS

Through our antimicrobial effectiveness studies, we realize that disinfectants do not kill all organisms. As all chemical agents may have an inherent bioburden (normally spores), we must assure that such bioburden is removed prior to their entry to our controlled areas. The transfer of such organisms through our disinfectants to our controlled areas, especially our aseptic filling areas, should be viewed as a catastrophic event. To even further reinforce the issue, we spread the disinfecting agents all over our walls, ceiling and floors. Controlling the contamination from ever entering is much easier that subsequently removing it from the controlled area. If we review regulatory expectations in this area we will find the requirement to sterilize all disinfectants and sporicides prior to entry to the controlled environment. The FDA has stated in its "Sterile Drug Products Produced by Aseptic Processing Draft" that, "Upon preparation, disinfectants should be rendered sterile, and used for a limited time, as specified by written procedures". Likewise, the European Union in EU Annex 1 states, "Disinfectants and detergents should be monitored for microbial contamination…". The Parenteral Drug Association's (PDA) Technical Report #70 states, "To ensure sanitizers, disinfectants, and sporicides do not represent a source of contamination, they should be sterile-filtered or sterilized before use in Grade A (ISO 5) and adjacent Grade B (ISO 5/6) areas."

Purchasing a disinfectant or sporicidal product as sterile from an audited vendor requires one to review the following critical items as a quality control measure to assure what one is using is sterile prior to use:

1. Assessment of the bioburden of the solution.
2. Assessment of the bioburden of the container that the solution is to be filled into.
3. Pre-washing containers (cleanliness level).
4. Requires a filter validation providing microorganisms are retained by the filter.
5. Assay of the solution (RTU or concentrate) to an acceptable active percentage.
6. Filtering the solution at 0.2 microns.
7. Aseptically filling the product into pre-sterilized containers or exposing the entire contents to a terminal sterilization process such as gamma irradiation.
8. Requires a lot-by-lot sterility test per current USP or EP compendium.
9. Conducting sterility testing requires the completion of *bacteriostasis* and *fungistasis* (B/F) testing. This proves that the sterility test is capable of growing organisms in the presence of the chemical agent.
10. Requires the assessment for expiration dating of an unopened container.

If the disinfectant or sporicide is to be processed sterile in-house, then the review of the following critical items as a quality control measure is suggested to assure what one is using is sterile prior to use:

1. Assessment of the bioburden of the solution.
2. Assessment of the bioburden of the container that the solution is to be filled into.
3. Pre-washing containers (cleanliness level).
4. Requires a filter validation providing microorganisms are retained by the filter.
5. Assay of the solution (RTU or concentrate) to an acceptable active percentage.
6. Filtering the solution at 0.2 microns.
7. Aseptically filling the product into pre-sterilized containers or exposing the entire contents to a terminal sterilization process such as gamma irradiation.

8. If the product is aseptically filtered, then the assurance that all that comes in contact with the product after the filter is rendered sterile.
9. Requires validation to be performed using a lot-by-lot sterility test per current USP or EP compendium or a bioburden analysis for at least three lots at the beginning and subsequently routinely tested as a quality control check. Sterility testing on a lot-by-lot basis need not be performed if sufficient validation testing is conducted.
10. Conducting sterility testing requires the completion of *bacteriostasis* and *fungistasis* (B/F) testing. This proves that the sterility test is capable of growing organisms in the presence of the chemical agent.
11. Requires the assessment for expiration dating of an unopened container.

Validation of our sterility claim for disinfectants should be a focus of our validation efforts. Normally the testing of three processed lots for sterility provides sufficient data. The pre-sterilization of our chemical agents prior to entry to the controlled area is simple common sense and common practice in the industry.

Container type is critical when using a sterile disinfectant. Container types include aerosol, trigger spray, squeeze bottle, and larger closed containers (one to five gallon and larger). Aerosol container is the most lucrative type, as the vessel does not aspirate the room air to the master reservoir. However, the container and its contents are required to be sterilized via gamma radiation or all the components pre-sterilized and subsequently filled via a validated aseptic filling operation. For obvious reasons, gamma sterilization of the entire contents is considered far superior methodology for achieving a sterile product. In 1992, the first sterile disinfectant, DECON AHOL® a sterile USP IPA, was marketed under US patent 6,123,900, Method of Sterilization. This patent and product showed the industry the effectiveness of this type of container. Thus, no viable or particulate contamination is returned to the solution contained. A pre-sterilized aerosol or pressurized vessel assures assay of the active ingredients (for the time period they remain stable) and sterility for the expiration period designated by the manufacturer.

Other smaller containers include the squeeze bottle and trigger spray bottles. While acceptable containers for all disinfectants and sporicides, the container itself aspirates the room air back to the master reservoir. Thus, assay and sterility are compromised after the initial use. The same is true for containers of one to five gallons and larger. Once opened sterility is compromised.

For varying disinfecting and sporicidal agents, a variety of containers need to be utilized. For ready-to-use mixtures we must decide how the product will be used. If in a smaller aerosol, trigger spray, or squeeze bottle, we may want to utilize a product that is pre-sterilized in this smaller form rather than attempting to pour or filter such solutions to an empty pre-sterilized container. We may also want to limit that the capping of product "to be used later" as our assay and sterility may be compromised over time. For concentrate products that need to be diluted with a quality water grade, we may want to look to implement unit-dose bottles that incorporate a pre-measured dose and are sterile. This system is superior to that of pouring a concentrate disinfectant or sporicide into a measuring cup and capping the remainder for later use. Questions may arise as to the assay and sterility of this remaining solution over time.

Thus, no viable or particulate contamination is returned to the solution contained. A pre-sterilized aerosol or pressurized vessel assures assay of the active ingredients (for the time period they remain stable) and sterility for the expiration period designated by the manufacturer.

3.10   AVAILABLE SANITIZERS, DISINFECTANTS, AND SPORICIDES FOR GMP OPERATION

The following chemical agents are the options for GMP operations. The choice is delineated by assessment of one's environmental flora derived over time and the compatibility of the agents with the surface substrates where they will be used.

Sanitizers:

- Isopropyl Alcohol 70%
- Ethanol at 70%
- Ethyl Alcohol at 70%
- Iodine (not normally used in clean room operations)

Disinfectants:

- Phenols
- Quaternary Ammonium
- Hydrogen Peroxide at 3% or below
- Sodium Hypochlorite below 0.10%

Sporicides/Sterilants:

- Sodium Hypochlorite above 0.25%
- Hydrogen Peroxide above 6% (sporicidal reduction at 6%)
- Peracetic Acid and Hydrogen Peroxide
- Glutaraldehyde
- Formaldehyde

In reviewing the basic types of chemical agents used in pharmaceutical and biotechnology operations we can come to understand their basic differences and applicability in our operations. To follow is a brief description of each of the most used chemical agents in the industry. As a complete chapter could be written on each, the summaries are brief, so we can develop a basic understanding of each chemical.

3.10.1   ISOPROPYL ALCOHOL, ETHYL ALCOHOL, ETHANOL SOLUTIONS

Alcohols have been used for years in pharmaceutical and biotechnology operations for three basic purposes: 1) as a sanitizing spray for gloves, surfaces, carts, etc.; 2) as a cleaning or wipe down agent to remove possible existent residues from critical non-product contact surfaces; and 3) as a product contact cleaning agent (ethyl alcohol only). In testing antimicrobial effectiveness of the products, a 70% solution demonstrates far superior efficacy performance than higher or lower concentrations. Alcohols come in a variety of forms. The most used forms in the clean room operation are isopropyl alcohol and ethyl alcohol (ethanol and alcohol). Over 90% of industry operation will utilize a 70% isopropyl alcohol solution to address clean room organisms as it has been proven more efficacious than ethyl alcohol (190–200 proof diluted to 70%) or ethanol (a mixture with the base as ethyl alcohol [63%] and spiked with methyl [3%] and isopropyl [4%]) at a small percentage (rendering it not drinkable). Alcohols demonstrate rapid broad spectrum antimicrobial activity against vegetative bacteria (including mycobacteria), viruses, and fungi but are not sporicidal. They are however, known to inhibit sporulation and spore germination, but this effect reversible. As alcohols are not sporicidal, they are not recommended for sterilization and are widely used for hard surface disinfection and skin antisepsis. As we have previously stated, of the existent alcohols, isopropyl alcohols demonstrate superior effectiveness against clean room organisms. However, for viruses, ethyl alcohol or ethanol seems to be slightly more effective and is used basically within the confines of the laboratory environment.

Published alcohol effectiveness or results of alcohol effectiveness are presented when sprayed to the surface and allowed to air dry. This should not be confused with the product's effectiveness if used in a saturated wipe. A saturated wipe contains a limited amount of the chemical agent. When used its dry times are significantly less, and thus, its destructive power substandard to that of the liquid itself on the surface. While the mechanism of wiping destroys cells in its action, the dry time of the alcohol is significantly faster.

Isopropyl alcohol wipes carry few if any claims. Usually they are used to wipe a surface in a cleaning operation (IPA wipe down) to remove existent disinfectant residues. Here also such products have a problem. As they are saturated with isopropyl alcohol, their ability to soak up residues and clean the surface is minimal. Most of the time these products just move the contamination around the surface. A superior methodology would be the use of an isopropyl alcohol and a dry wipe. Like cleaning a window, we would spray the solution to the surface and wipe. This will remove most of the contaminants on the surface. This can be proven in a home experiment by using a saturated wipe to clean a window. When completed, the window will have streaks, or swirls and look as though the dirt was just moved around. If one were to conduct the same experiment with a dry wipe and spray isopropyl alcohol, the surface would appear much cleaner. The soaking of the liquid with contaminants in suspension from the surface into a dry wipe is a superior methodology. During isopropyl alcohol wipe downs of non-product contact but critical surfaces, we need to employ the cleaner of the two methodologies. Rendering of the products as sterile is a must prior to use in a Class 100 (Grade A and B, ISO 5) and adjacent Class 10,000 (Grade C, ISO 7) areas. Sterilization of disinfection agents is discussed in depth in this chapter in section 3.9: Sterility of Disinfecting Agents.

3.10.2 PHENOLS

Phenolics have been used for years as a disinfecting agent. Phenolics are effective against gram-positive and gram-negative organisms. However, phenols exhibit better antimicrobial effectiveness against gram-positive organisms than they do against gram-negative organisms. They have limited activity against fungi and certain virus strains such as HIV-1 (AIDS virus) and Herpes Simplex, Type 2. Phenolics normally are available in an alkaline and acid base version. The theory surrounding the rotation of these two compounds is described later in the chapter. Overall, phenolics demonstrate superior antimicrobial effectiveness in an acidic base as opposed to an alkaline base. Some of the most common chemical compounds in phenolic germicidal detergents are in a low pH phenolic: an ortho-phenyl-phenol and ortho-benzyl-benzyl-para-chlorophenol and in a high pH phenolic: a sodium ortho-benzyl-para-chlorophenate, sodium ortho-phenylphenate, or sodium para-tertiary-amylphenate. While phenols provide good broad spectrum disinfection, they are not sporicidal and have major drawbacks in their use. One drawback is the horrific residues that are noticed from long-term use of the products. Phenolics are normally an amber or light tan color when manufactured. This color darkens with age and its exposure to light (especially fluorescent). Residues start as a "dripping droplet" that is not easily removed. The use of 70% isopropyl alcohol or certain residue removers can remove such residues in their early existence on surfaces. While somewhat effective, both residue-cleaning products eventually give way to the darkening phenolic that stains the surface with a dark brown color. Transfer of such residues to an unwanted location is a concern and precautionary measures need to be implemented to assure minimization of this scenario. Compatibility with most chemicals is normally very good, however, the effect of anionic characteristic of the chemical in relation to applications in conjunction with a cationic surfactant such as a quaternary ammonium has been reported as problematic. Expiration of a formulated phenol also carries some concern. The formulation in a closed container should remain stable for a seven- to 30-day period (dependent upon storage). Formulated solutions should be marked accordingly. The normality in the industry is seven days and less if the solution is in an open container (such as a bucket) and should be discarded each day. Rendering of these products as sterile is a must prior to use in a Class 100 (Grade A and B, ISO 5) and adjacent Class 10,000 (Grade C, ISO 7) areas. Sterilization of disinfection agents is discussed in depth in section 3.9: Sterility of Disinfecting Agents.

3.10.3   QUATERNARY AMMONIUM COMPOUNDS

Quaternary ammonium products are used in more disinfection applications than phenolic germicidal detergents. Their spectrum of use is very broad and ranges throughout the industrial world, through hospital and institutional settings and even home use. Quaternary ammoniums have excellent detergency. They are one of the best cleaners among the spectrum of disinfecting agents. These cationic solutions also have excellent deodorizing capabilities. Quaternary ammonium compounds are effective against gram-positive and gram-negative organisms. However, phenols exhibit better antimicrobial effectiveness against gram-positive organisms than they do against gram-negative organisms. They have limited activity against fungi and certain virus strains such as HIV-1 (AIDS virus) and Herpes Simplex, Type 2. In fact, and due to competition in this arena, quaternary ammonium compounds have the most organisms registered as label claims with the US EPA. Their mechanism of antimicrobial effectiveness is related to their positively charged molecule. Simply, the positively charged molecule attracts to the negatively charged microorganism's cell wall. The cycle of kill is complete when the chemical agent is absorbed into the cell and spread throughout the organism. Quaternary ammoniums are available in both alkaline and acid-based compounds. Quaternary ammonium compounds normally utilize an alkyl dimethyl benzyl ammonium chloride or a dimethyl ethyl benzyl ammonium chloride. While a multitude of formulations exist in the industry, these are two of the most popular components. As with phenols, quaternary ammoniums do leave sticky residues that become problematic over time. However, they are not of the scale of phenolic residues. Expiration of a formulated (from concentrate) quaternary ammonium also carries some concern. The formulation in a closed container is relatively stable and should remain stable for a 30-day period in a closed container. Formulated solutions should be marked accordingly. The normality in the industry is seven to 30 days and less if the solution is in an open container (such as a bucket) and should be discarded each day. However, in recent years, quaternary ammoniums have been made in ready-to-use formulas that are very stable. Rendering of these products as sterile is a must prior to use in a Class 100 (Grade A and B, ISO 5) and adjacent Class 10,000 (Grade C, ISO 7) areas. Sterilization of disinfection agents is discussed in depth in this chapter in section 3.9: Sterility of Disinfecting Agents.

3.10.4 SODIUM HYPOCHLORITE

Sodium hypochlorite solutions are one of the oldest known disinfectants and sporicidal agents. The product is available in many forms including ready-to-use 0.25% and 0.52% solution, to concentrate 5.25% and 10% solutions, to powders that are mixed with water to formulate a variety of solutions. Bleach as we know it is normally found in a 5.25% concentration, however, in recent years such formulations from the Clorox Corporation® have been increase to a near 7% solution to assure continued stability of the active percentage.

One of the main problems with the use of sodium hypochlorite is that it is used at too strong of an active percentage. Sodium hypochlorite is used throughout the healthcare setting and normally diluted to concentrations of 0.25 or 0.52%. One of the problems with sodium hypochlorite formulations is the method of formulation designation that varies from firm to firm. Some formulate to a part per million (ppm), some to a percentage of a solution and some to a dilution such as 1–10. At a use-dilution of 0.25% (or a 1–20 dilution or 250 ppm) sodium hypochlorite is effective against gram-positive and gram-negative organisms, viruses, fungi, and bacterial endospores. At a slightly increased use-dilution of 0.52% (or a 1–10 dilution or 500 ppm) sodium hypochlorite is effective against gram-positive and gram-negative organisms, viruses, fungi, and more effective against a wider range of bacterial endospores. Both formulations are used throughout the pharmaceutical and biotechnology industry.

In formulation of a sodium hypochlorite solution, many chose to acidify the solution that makes it a more potent mixture when focusing on bacterial endospores. However, acidification causes rapid degradation of the active elements in the solution and use of the product is limited to approximately two hours. Acidification may not be necessary as the product demonstrates excellent sporicidal characteristics in its neutral state and bacterial endospore levels in clean rooms are not exuberant in numbers (above 1.0×10^6) and there is no soil load. A formulation of 250 or 500 ppm has excellent sporicidal activity. However, expiration of the solution can become a problem. A normal 5.25% concentrate sodium hypochlorite normally carries a one-year expiration for an unopened container. Some companies have validated and increased this expiration with applicable assay data over time to 18 months. Once opened, whether in a ready-to-use formula or a concentrate product, the product needs to be used within a 30-day period. Open containers (such as buckets, and open bottles) have a shorter expiration as the chlorine in the solution begins to burn off leaving only the sodium chloride. Open containers should be formulated and used within the same day.

Some drawbacks with sodium hypochlorite are mainly focused on the residue and corrosiveness of the product. As previously stated, the chlorine in the solution begins to burn off leaving only the sodium chloride. This white crystal-like residue attacks the impurities in stainless steel (as an example) over a longer time frame. When using a sodium hypochlorite solution, it is imperative to remove the sodium chloride residues frequently to minimize this corrosive action. Rendering of these products as sterile is a must prior to use in a Class 100 (Grade A and B, ISO 5) and adjacent Class 10,000 (Grade C, ISO 7) areas. Sterilization of disinfection agents is discussed in depth in section 3.9: Sterility of Disinfecting Agents.

3.10.5 HYDROGEN PEROXIDE

Hydrogen peroxide is one of the most common disinfectants in the industrial marketplace. The product is commonly used as an antiseptic in hospitals or for consumer use at a 3% solution. In the pharmaceutical and biotechnology industry, hydrogen peroxide is used at 35% as a sterilant in isolators and at 3–10% for surface disinfection. Dependent upon the concentration used, hydrogen peroxide is effective against bacteria, yeasts, viruses, and bacterial spores. Destruction of spores is greatly increased both with a rise in temperature and increase in concentration. Hydrogen peroxide is a clear, colorless liquid that is environmentally friendly as it can rapidly degrade into water and oxygen. While generally stable, most hydrogen peroxide formulations contain a preservative to prevent decomposition. At lower concentrations (3–10%) the chemical is effective against gram-positive and gram-negative bacteria, viruses, and bacterial endospores in lower enumerations. However, at higher concentrations and longer contact times the product exhibits superior sporicidal reduction of bacterial spores. Some of the positive features of the product are its mild, if any, odor and its low residue characteristics. However, the product also has some setbacks in exceeding OSHA exposure limits if used in confinement in too large a quantity. Precautions should be taken for its use. Rendering of these products as sterile is a must prior to use in a Class 100 (Grade A and B, ISO 5) and adjacent Class 10,000 (Grade C, ISO 7) areas. Sterilization of disinfection agents is discussed in depth in section 3.9: Sterility of Disinfecting Agents.

3.10.6 PERACETIC ACID AND HYDROGEN PEROXIDE

Peracetic acid and hydrogen peroxide mixtures have received much recent attention in the pharmaceutical and biotechnology industry in recent years. The chemical is considered a more potent biocide than hydrogen peroxide being bactericidal, virucidal, fungicidal, and sporicidal at very low concentrations (<0.3%). The product was originally designed for the sterilization of medical devices. The chemical destroys the cell by destroying vital membrane lipids, DNA and denatures proteins, and enzymes. Peracetic acid and hydrogen peroxide mixtures decompose to acetic acid and oxygen. Active percentages of marketed products range from 0.3% to 1.3% as a sterilant in both ready-to-use and concentrate solutions. Ready-to-use solutions require a very high level of acetic acid as a stabilizer, nearing 5.2%. While concentrate products need smaller amounts of acetic acid in the formulation. Concentrate solutions incorporate approximately 8% acetic acid and upon formulation to a use-dilution, this value drops to near 0.4%.

One of the main misconceptions with the use of peracetic acid and hydrogen peroxide mixtures as well as most registered sporicides is that the product needs to be used at the sterilant label claim active percentage. First, we must understand the requirements set for by the EPA. The EPA requires all registrants making label claims to do so by following test methods outlined in AOAC protocol. The sterilant claim on products/labels follows the AOAC sporicidal test. This test requires the complete reduction of 10^6 of *B. subtilis* and *C. sporogenes* in a 60-carrier test, at 20°C, in a soil load. In the clean room, bioburden is significantly lower. Thus, the active percentage needed to destroy the flora normally seen is significantly less. Simply, registered sterilant label claims are too strong for what is noticed in a clean room. Coupled with the high enumeration of the AOAC test parameters are also a soil load, not present in clean rooms. Thus, end users should look to validate a concentration of peracetic acid and hydrogen peroxide mixtures as well as other registered sporicides at realistic bioburden values as discussed later in this chapter in the section Determining Antimicrobial Effectiveness. This will significantly reduce odors, deterioration of surfaces, problematic user situations, and residues.

Peracetic acid and hydrogen peroxide mixtures have a pungent vinegar smell that is offensive, if not intolerable to many users. Due to the horrific smell and the characteristic drying of mucosal membranes, peracetic acid and hydrogen peroxide mixtures have dissatisfaction among end users. Facilities that have used sodium hypochlorite (bleach) for years find the transition to peracetic acid and hydrogen peroxide very difficult in terms of worker satisfaction. The product, if used in a clean room environment that may have 15–20% fresh air, may easily exceed required levels when industrial hygiene testing is performed. Safety precautions for end users should be assured prior to its use. While reports of the product deem it non-corrosive to metals, industry reports have shown this product reacts adversely with most stainless steels, aluminums, plastics, epoxies, and most clean room surfaces. After application, a white cloudy residue is normally left that requires either an IPA wipe down or a water-for-injection (WFI) rinse to remove.

3.10.7 GLUTARALDEHYDE

Glutaraldehyde has been used for some time as a disinfectant and sterilant for endoscopes and surgical equipment. Glutaraldehyde is normally sold in a 2.0% solution. The product is usually supplied as an amber solution with an acid pH. Glutaraldehyde is a powerful biocidal agent having the advantage of continued activity in the presence of organic material. Glutaraldehyde has broad spectrum activity against bacteria, bacterial spores, viruses, and fungi. The mechanism of action involves the destruction of the outer layers of the cell. Glutaraldehyde is the only aldehyde to exhibit excellent sporicidal activity. In recent years, glutaraldehyde's use has been focused mainly on the hospital environment. Many pharmaceutical and biotechnology organizations do not use a glutaraldehyde product in their operations. The product is very toxic and specific handling precautions must be employed prior to its use. Especially noted are the gaseous fumes and the possible absorption through human tissue (skin).

3.10.8 FORMALDEHYDE

Formaldehyde is widely known as a fumigant for rooms and buildings. It has been shown to be effective against bacteria and bacteria spores and vegetative bacteria. Acklund et al. (1980) showed that at 20°C and a relative humidity of approximately 100%, a six-log reduction of *B. subtilis* spores was obtained after one and a half hours exposure to 300 µ/L whereas at 250 µg/L only a four-log reduction was obtained after six hours of exposure. The mechanism of action of formaldehyde is assumed to be due to the reaction with cell protein and DNA or RNA (Russell, 1976).

Formaldehyde is normally used in the pharmaceutical and the biotechnology industry to bring back an area after shutting down or major maintenance. During its implementation very stringent safety precautions are assured for personnel protection that include areas and building clearance and hold times of areas prior to release.

While formaldehyde is effective, this chapter has focused on routine methods of cleaning and disinfection. Formaldehyde does not fit appropriately as a choice in this venue and would be used as a mechanism in opening a new area or as a method when coming back from a shutdown period.

3.11 ANTIMICROBIAL EFFECTIVENESS TESTING CONDUCTED ON GMP ENVIRONMENTAL ISOLATES AND ATCC CULTURES AT VAI LABORATORIES

Most GMP regulatory inspectors will look at the product label claims and say to the GMP firm, "Have you verified this efficacy using your isolates on your clean room substrates?" When first hearing this many GMP firms will want to push back until they realize what the inspector is asking is what the antimicrobial registering body does not include in their requirements to register the product. The first discrepancy is related to specific isolates recovered from the GMP facility to show that the agent being utilized can adequately destroy the organism. The second discrepancy is the dry time or contact time that was used in the approval of the antimicrobial agent with the antimicrobial agent registering body. Most probably for a disinfectant this was ten minutes and for a sporicide/sterilant it could have been hours. This difference is related to the population each body feels should be destroyed by the antimicrobial agent. A government agency like the US EPA would want to see minimally one million CFUs or a 1.0×10^6 population destroyed by the agent in the contact time prescribed. However, in no GMP firm would such bioburden exist and so while the GMP regulatory inspector wants to see a faster time for efficacy they also agree the bioburden should be less from 1,000 CFUs (1.0×10^4) to 10,000 CFUs (1.0×10^5). Nor would surfaces have a dry time or contact time for the agent on the surface for that length of time. This time period would be much shorter nearing 30–60 seconds for alcohol-based products and three to five minutes for water-based products. The third discrepancy related to the carrier surface the test was performed on. For an AOAC test to meet many authorities such as the US EPA or Australian TGA, ceramic penicylinders are used and sporicidal sutures are also employed. There are very few firms that would have ceramic as a surface substrate or would the need to know the efficacy on sutures. However, a hospital would desire this information, and this is where worldwide antimicrobial agent registration has its basis. Clean room substrates defined earlier in this chapter represent what we would expect to see in GMP operations and a GMP firm needs to know the expected antimicrobial effectiveness of agents on such surfaces that inherently have such bioburden.

As testing commences the GMP laboratory professional must also take into account realistic attributes of what he or she is doing. Your goal is to provide useful data that can be utilized in operations. In reality, you are performing a lab study on a coupon that measures anywhere from $1'' \times 0.5''$ to $2'' \times 2''$. On that coupon will be 10^4–10^5 of an organism. The surface size is not depictive of a clean room surface that will be disinfected. The enumeration of microorganisms is not representative of the flora which will be noticed on any surface in any area in your facility. In fact, the enumeration is outrageously high. On the surface you test will be no residues and very little particulate that would characterize your areas. You are applying the agent perfectly which might not be done day after day. You are not wiping or mopping which will surely remove more contamination from the surface. In short, it is a very controlled experiment in the lab that does not take into account personnel training in cleaning and disinfection nor SOPs that will need to be written. It is important to understand that what you are doing is extreme overkill and what you assess in acceptance criteria should be realistic. Realistic acceptance criteria is > one log per PDA Technical report #70. In that first log you will have destroyed 90% of the inoculate. A second and third log of reduction are miniscule compared to what you attained in the first log. And by requiring the second and/or third log you most probably have invoked much higher residuals in your facility and placed cleaning personnel potentially into a higher vapor cleaning scenario. And, in doing so have not really increased the efficacy performance to any value that matters as the extra strength was not required. All that you are doing needs to be scientifically assessed and assured that it can be repeated day-in and day-out in operations.

Many times, quality professionals possibly think too much about the testing scenario and forget about what will happen in operations. Imagine being part of the cleaning crew. For our example I will use paint as the chemical agent and brushes and rollers as our mops and wipers. Each day you come in and say to your manager "What are we going to do today?" The manager's response is "We are going to paint the room". So the manager gives you paint brushes, rollers, paint, and tape. And you do a great job painting the room making sure you remove outlet covers, light switches, tape windows, etc. The next day you come in you ask the same question, and the response if the same. So again, you do a fantastic job painting the room cause the manager must want two coats. The next day and for the following 100 days the manager responds to the question with the same answer, "We are going to paint the room". Now you are frustrated, bored and the repetition is ridiculous. So each time you do not do as good a job because the next day you will have to do the same thing, paint the room. At day 300, you miss the left wall, you paint over top of the windows and your sense of perfection is definitely lacking. This is what it is like being part of the cleaning crew. To add to your joy, they make you wear gowns that cause you to sweat. Your goggles fog constantly and the vapors from the chemicals dry your nose and you smell the smell even after you are home for the evening. This is what being part of the cleaning crew is like and no antimicrobial effectiveness testing (AET) study or validation study can prepare an operation for this type of scenario. So it is lost, forgotten but it is the thing that causes problematic environmental situations, as contamination that was let in has a flawed corrective action. So when we assess stringent acceptance criteria, we further complicate this scenario as corrosion occurs, disinfection is done more quickly and residues are left remaining. It is food for thought to take yourself out of quality assurance or validation and imagine yourself in production services.

So, what will the GMP firm expect to see in antimicrobial effectiveness results. For over 25 years VAI Laboratories have assisted GMP firms with the antimicrobial effectiveness testing. The results presented represent results from lab studies for varying agents against varying organisms on varying surfaces at varying dry time or contact times.

Disclaimer: The following test report and the data contained therein is not intended to, and does not have any relationship to, nor does it amend or is intended to amend any information contained in any labels or registrations required or approved by the United States Environmental Protection Agency (EPA) or any state pursuant to any law, including but not limited to the Federal Insecticide, Fungicide, and Rodenticide Act (7 USC Sections 136 et seq), or any state analog, or any other foreign or international legal body or jurisdiction, for the antimicrobial agents utilized and referenced in the study. The data presented represents a private testing study and regimen ("Study") that investigated solely "whether microorganisms could be destroyed on carrier surfaces, as tested at lower populations which would depict bioburden in the clean room, and shorter contact or dry times, which is depictive of the GMP setting and an expectation by regulatory agencies such as the US Food and Drug Administration (FDA)." Prior to use of any product containing such chemical germicides or antimicrobial agents which are referenced and/or used in the study, all persons are advised by this Disclaimer to review all applicable labels and registrations associated with each such product.

Peracetic Acid and H$_2$O$_2$ in WFI				
Organism Tested	Surface	Wetted Period	Initial Positive Control Inoculate	Results in Log Reduction
Bacillus subtilis	Stainless Steel	5	5.50×10^4	4.74
Aspergillus brasiliensis	Stainless Steel	5	5.15×10^4	2.49
Staphylococcus aureus	Stainless Steel	5	3.60×10^4	4.56
Pseudomonas aeruginosa	Stainless Steel	5	2.74×10^4	4.44
Candida albicans	Stainless Steel	5	1.48×10^4	5.17
Micrococcus luteus	Stainless Steel	5	4.55×10^4	4.66
Penicillium rubens	Stainless Steel	5	5.80×10^4	4.76
Bacillus cereus	Stainless Steel	5	1.15×10^3	1.54
Cladosporium cladosporioides	Stainless Steel	5	2.15×10^4	4.33
Penicillium glabrum	Stainless Steel	5	1.39×10^4	4.14
Bacillus subtilis	Stainless Steel	10	5.50×10^4	4.74
Aspergillus brasiliensis	Stainless Steel	10	5.15×10^4	3.49
Staphylococcus aureus	Stainless Steel	10	3.60×10^4	4.56
Pseudomonas aeruginosa	Stainless Steel	10	2.74×10^4	4.44
Candida albicans	Stainless Steel	10	1.48×10^4	5.17
Micrococcus luteus	Stainless Steel	10	4.55×10^4	4.66
Penicillium rubens	Stainless Steel	10	5.80×10^4	4.79
Bacillus cereus	Stainless Steel	10	1.15×10^3	3.06
Cladosporium cladosporioides	Stainless Steel	10	2.15×10^4	4.33
Penicillium glabrum	Stainless Steel	10	1.39×10^4	4.14
Bacillus subtilis	Epoxy	5	7.70×10^4	4.89
Aspergillus brasiliensis	Epoxy	5	5.05×10^4	2.88
Staphylococcus aureus	Epoxy	5	3.90×10^4	4.59
Pseudomonas aeruginosa	Epoxy	5	2.55×10^4	4.41
Candida albicans	Epoxy	5	1.50×10^5	5.18
Micrococcus luteus	Epoxy	5	5.10×10^4	4.71
Penicillium rubens	Epoxy	5	6.50×10^4	4.85
Bacillus cereus	Epoxy	5	1.55×10^3	1.12
Cladosporium cladosporioides	Epoxy	5	1.54×10^4	4.19
Penicillium glabrum	Epoxy	5	9.55×10^3	3.98
Bacillus subtilis	Epoxy	10	7.70×10^4	4.89
Aspergillus brasiliensis	Epoxy	10	5.05×10^4	2.78
Staphylococcus aureus	Epoxy	10	3.90×10^4	4.59
Pseudomonas aeruginosa	Epoxy	10	2.55×10^4	4.41
Candida albicans	Epoxy	10	1.50×10^5	5.18
Micrococcus luteus	Epoxy	10	5.10×10^4	4.71
Penicillium rubens	Epoxy	10	6.50×10^4	4.85
Bacillus cereus	Epoxy	10	1.55×10^3	1.97
Cladosporium cladosporioides	Epoxy	10	1.54×10^4	4.19
Penicillium glabrum	Epoxy	10	9.55×10^3	3.98

70% Isopropyl Alcohol in WFI				
Organism Tested	Surface	Wetted Period	Initial Positive Control Inoculate	Results in Log Reduction
Micrococcus luteus	Stainless Steel	30s	1.53×10^4	4.18
Staphylococcus aureus	Stainless Steel	30s	1.13×10^5	3.83
Pseudomonas aeruginosa	Stainless Steel	30s	3.10×10^5	4.27
Staphylococcus epidermidis	Stainless Steel	30s	1.19×10^6	3.63
Staphylococcus warneri	Stainless Steel	30s	1.02×10^5	3.49
Kocuria polaris	Stainless Steel	30s	9.50×10^3	3.94
Staphylococcus hominis	Stainless Steel	30s	4.25×10^4	3.11
Coryebacterium aurimucosum	Stainless Steel	30s	1.08×10^5	5.03
Penicillium chrysogenum	Stainless Steel	30s	1.39×10^6	3.33
Neurospora crassa	Stainless Steel	30s	9.40×10^4	3.05
Micrococcus luteus	Stainless Steel	60s	1.53×10^4	4.18
Staphylococcus aureus	Stainless Steel	60s	1.13×10^5	4.56
Pseudomonas aeruginosa	Stainless Steel	60s	3.10×10^5	5.49
Staphylococcus epidermidis	Stainless Steel	60s	1.19×10^6	3.63
Staphylococcus warneri	Stainless Steel	60s	1.02×10^5	3.19
Kocuria polaris	Stainless Steel	60s	9.50×10^3	6.00
Staphylococcus hominis	Stainless Steel	60s	4.25×10^4	4.63
Coryebacterium aurimucosum	Stainless Steel	60s	1.08×10^5	5.03
Penicillium chrysogenum	Stainless Steel	60s	1.39×10^6	3.60
Neurospora crassa	Stainless Steel	60s	9.40×10^4	2.87
Micrococcus luteus	Nitrile Glove	30s	1.56×10^5	1.95
Staphylococcus epidermidis	Nitrile Glove	30s	2.06×10^4	1.88
Staphylococcus warneri	Nitrile Glove	30s	2.21×10^5	2.05
Kocuria polaris	Nitrile Glove	30s	1.02×10^6	5.09
Staphylococcus hominis	Nitrile Glove	30s	4.15×10^4	4.62
Coryebacterium aurimucosum	Nitrile Glove	30s	1.07×10^5	5.03
Penicillium chrysogenum	Nitrile Glove	30s	1.50×10^5	2.54
Neurospora crassa	Nitrile Glove	30s	1.13×10^5	2.29
Micrococcus luteus	Nitrile Glove	60s	1.56×10^5	2.3
Staphylococcus epidermidis	Nitrile Glove	60s	2.06×10^4	2.61
Staphylococcus warneri	Nitrile Glove	60s	2.21×10^5	3.08
Kocuria polaris	Nitrile Glove	60s	1.02×10^6	6.01
Staphylococcus hominis	Nitrile Glove	60s	4.15×10^4	4.62
Coryebacterium aurimucosum	Nitrile Glove	60s	1.07×10^5	5.03
Penicillium chrysogenum	Nitrile Glove	60s	1.50×10^5	2.54
Neurospora crassa	Nitrile Glove	60s	1.13×10^5	2.56

70% Ethanol in WFI

Organism Tested	Surface	Wetted Period	Initial Positive Control Inoculate	Results in Log Reduction
Staphylococcus aureus	Stainless Steel	30s	6.60×10^4	4.82
Escherichia coli	Stainless Steel	30s	2.17×10^4	4.34
Pseudomonas aeruginosa	Stainless Steel	30s	9.20×10^4	4.96
Micrococcus luteus	Stainless Steel	30s	1.17×10^4	4.07
Staphylococcus aureus	Stainless Steel	60s	2.31×10^4	3.14
Escherichia coli	Stainless Steel	60s	2.17×10^4	3.12
Pseudomonas aeruginosa	Stainless Steel	60s	9.20×10^4	3.44
Micrococcus luteus	Stainless Steel	60s	1.17×10^4	4.07

High pH Phenol in WFI

Organism Tested	Surface	Wetted Period	Initial Positive Control Inoculate	Results in Log Reduction
Pseudomonas aeruginosa	Stainless Steel	5 min	6.10×10^3	3.79
Staphylococcus aureus	Stainless Steel	5 min	1.06×10^6	6.03
Bacillus subtilis	Stainless Steel	5 min	2.29×10^4	1.74
Escherichia coli	Stainless Steel	5 min	2.00×10^5	5.3
Aspergillus brasiliensis	Stainless Steel	5 min	1.53×10^6	3.11
Candida albicans	Stainless Steel	5 min	1.23×10^4	4.09
Clostridium sporogenes	Stainless Steel	5 min	1.74×10^4	2.72
Micrococcus luteus	Stainless Steel	5 min	1.35×10^5	5.13
Bacillus cereus	Stainless Steel	5 min	6.00×10^5	6.56
Staphylococcus epidermidis	Stainless Steel	5 min	3.65×10^6	3.54
Pseudomonas aeruginosa	Stainless Steel	10 min	6.10×10^3	3.79
Staphylococcus aureus	Stainless Steel	10 min	1.06×10^6	6.03
Bacillus subtilis	Stainless Steel	10 min	2.29×10^4	1.76
Escherichia coli	Stainless Steel	10 min	2.00×10^5	4.08
Aspergillus brasiliensis	Stainless Steel	10 min	1.53×10^6	3.81
Candida albicans	Stainless Steel	10 min	1.23×10^4	4.09
Clostridium sporogenes	Stainless Steel	10 min	1.74×10^4	2.54
Micrococcus luteus	Stainless Steel	10 min	1.35×10^5	5.13
Bacillus cereus	Stainless Steel	10 min	6.00×10^5	6.56
Staphylococcus epidermidis	Stainless Steel	10 min	3.65×10^6	3.65
Pseudomonas aeruginosa	Epoxy	5 min	6.20×10^3	3.79
Staphylococcus aureus	Epoxy	5 min	1.08×10^5	6.03
Bacillus subtilis	Epoxy	5 min	2.23×10^4	1.6
Escherichia coli	Epoxy	5 min	2.07×10^5	3.31
Aspergillus brasiliensis	Epoxy	5 min	1.72×10^6	2.57

Candida albicans	Epoxy	5 min	1.21×10^4	4.08
Clostridium sporogenes	Epoxy	5 min	1.83×10^4	1.89
Micrococcus luteus	Epoxy	5 min	1.35×10^5	5.13
Bacillus cereus	Epoxy	5 min	6.00×10^5	5.56
Staphylococcus epidermidis	Epoxy	5 min	3.65×10^6	3.57
Pseudomonas aeruginosa	Epoxy	10 min	6.20×10^3	2.57
Staphylococcus aureus	Epoxy	10 min	1.08×10^5	6.03
Bacillus subtilis	Epoxy	10 min	2.23×10^4	1.47
Escherichia coli	Epoxy	10 min	2.07×10^5	5.31
Aspergillus brasiliensis	Epoxy	10 min	1.72×10^6	3.24
Candida albicans	Epoxy	10 min	1.21×10^4	4.08
Clostridium sporogenes	Epoxy	10 min	1.83×10^4	1.68
Micrococcus luteus	Epoxy	10 min	1.35×10^5	5.13
Bacillus cereus	Epoxy	10 min	6.00×10^5	6.56
Staphylococcus epidermidis	Epoxy	10 min	3.65×10^6	3.62

Low pH Phenol in WFI

Organism Tested	Surface	Wetted Period	Initial Positive Control Inoculate	Results in Log Reduction
Staphylococcus aureus	Stainless Steel	5 min	2.70×10^6	4.73
Pseudomonas aeruginosa	Stainless Steel	5 min	8.15×10^6	5.21
Candida albicans	Stainless Steel	5 min	2.66×10^6	4.72
Aspergillus brasiliensis	Stainless Steel	5 min	1.61×10^5	2.30
Penicillium citrinum	Stainless Steel	5 min	1.83×10^5	3.56
Penicillium glabrum	Stainless Steel	5 min	1.56×10^5	3.49
Bacillus licheniformis	Stainless Steel	5 min	2.30×10^4	0.49
Micrococcus luteus	Stainless Steel	5 min	3.40×10^4	4.53
Bacillus subtilis	Stainless Steel	5 min	1.90×10^4	2.36
Brevibacillus borstelensis	Stainless Steel	5 min	6.10×10^4	1.91
Staphylococcus aureus	Stainless Steel	10 min	2.70×10^6	4.73
Pseudomonas aeruginosa	Stainless Steel	10 min	8.15×10^6	5.09
Candida albicans	Stainless Steel	10 min	2.66×10^6	4.72
Aspergillus brasiliensis	Stainless Steel	10 min	1.61×10^5	2.73
Penicillium citrinum	Stainless Steel	10 min	1.83×10^5	3.56
Penicillium glabrum	Stainless Steel	10 min	1.56×10^5	3.49
Bacillus licheniformis	Stainless Steel	10 min	2.30×10^4	0.62
Micrococcus luteus	Stainless Steel	10 min	3.40×10^4	4.56
Bacillus subtilis	Stainless Steel	10 min	1.90×10^4	2.28
Brevibacillus borstelensis	Stainless Steel	10 min	6.10×10^4	2.27
Staphylococcus aureus	Epoxy	5 min	3.75×10^6	4.50
Pseudomonas aeruginosa	Epoxy	5 min	7.20×10^7	3.99

Candida albicans	Epoxy	5 min	2.70×10^6	3.17
Aspergillus brasiliensis	Epoxy	5 min	1.25×10^5	1.57
Penicillium citrinum	Epoxy	5 min	1.48×10^5	1.78
Penicillium glabrum	Epoxy	5 min	1.71×10^5	2.20
Bacillus licheniformis	Epoxy	5 min	3.00×10^4	0.64
Micrococcus luteus	Epoxy	5 min	4.00×10^4	4.60
Bacillus subtilis	Epoxy	5 min	8.50×10^3	1.59
Brevibacillus borstelensis	Epoxy	5 min	5.60×10^4	1.23
Staphylococcus aureus	Epoxy	10 min	3.75×10^6	4.87
Pseudomonas aeruginosa	Epoxy	10 min	7.20×10^7	3.78
Candida albicans	Epoxy	10 min	2.70×10^6	3.34
Aspergillus brasiliensis	Epoxy	10 min	1.25×10^5	1.87
Penicillium citrinum	Epoxy	10 min	1.48×10^5	2.39
Penicillium glabrum	Epoxy	10 min	1.71×10^5	3.16
Bacillus licheniformis	Epoxy	10 min	3.00×10^4	0.76
Micrococcus luteus	Epoxy	10 min	4.00×10^4	4.60
Bacillus subtilis	Epoxy	10 min	8.50×10^3	1.33
Brevibacillus borstelensis	Epoxy	10 min	5.60×10^4	1.17

Quaternary Ammonium in WFI

Organism Tested	Surface	Wetted Period	Initial Positive Control Inoculate	Results in Log Reduction
Aspergillus brasiliensis	Stainless Steel	5 min	4.60×10^4	4.66
Staphylococcus aureus	Stainless Steel	5 min	8.20×10^4	4.91
Pseudomonas aeruginosa	Stainless Steel	5 min	3.85×10^4	4.59
Candida albicans	Stainless Steel	5 min	1.31×10^4	4.12
Micrococcus luteus	Stainless Steel	5 min	1.10×10^4	4.04
Penicillium rubens	Stainless Steel	5 min	9.05×10^4	4.96
Bacillus subtilis	Stainless Steel	5 min	1.34×10^4	1.25
Staphylococcus epidermidis	Stainless Steel	5 min	2.16×10^4	4.33
Escherichia coli	Stainless Steel	5 min	2.00×10^5	5.36
Clostridium sporogenes	Stainless Steel	5 min	1.74×10^4	2.72
Aspergillus brasiliensis	Stainless Steel	10 min	4.60×10^4	4.66
Staphylococcus aureus	Stainless Steel	10 min	8.20×10^4	4.91
Pseudomonas aeruginosa	Stainless Steel	10 min	3.85×10^4	4.59
Candida albicans	Stainless Steel	10 min	1.31×10^4	4.12
Micrococcus luteus	Stainless Steel	10 min	1.10×10^4	4.04
Penicillium rubens	Stainless Steel	10 min	9.05×10^4	4.96
Bacillus subtilis	Stainless Steel	10 min	1.34×10^4	1.59
Staphylococcus epidermidis	Stainless Steel	10 min	2.16×10^4	4.33
Escherichia coli	Stainless Steel	10 min	2.00×10^5	4.08

Clostridium sporogenes	Stainless Steel	10 min	1.74×10^4	2.54
Aspergillus brasiliensis	Epoxy	5 min	5.65×10^4	4.75
Staphylococcus aureus	Epoxy	5 min	6.80×10^4	4.83
Pseudomonas aeruginosa	Epoxy	5 min	5.15×10^4	4.71
Candida albicans	Epoxy	5 min	1.31×10^4	4.12
Micrococcus luteus	Epoxy	5 min	1.26×10^4	4.10
Penicillium rubens	Epoxy	5 min	7.60×10^4	4.88
Bacillus subtilis	Epoxy	5 min	1.61×10^4	1.20
Staphylococcus epidermidis	Epoxy	5 min	1.90×10^4	4.28
Escherichia coli	Epoxy	5 min	2.07×10^4	3.31
Clostridium sporogenes	Epoxy	5 min	1.83×10^4	1.89
Aspergillus brasiliensis	Epoxy	10 min	5.65×10^4	3.23
Staphylococcus aureus	Epoxy	10 min	6.80×10^4	4.83
Pseudomonas aeruginosa	Epoxy	10 min	5.15×10^4	4.71
Candida albicans	Epoxy	10 min	1.31×10^4	4.12
Micrococcus luteus	Epoxy	10 min	1.26×10^4	4.1
Penicillium rubens	Epoxy	10 min	7.60×10^4	4.88
Bacillus subtilis	Epoxy	10 min	1.61×10^4	1.33
Staphylococcus epidermidis	Epoxy	10 min	1.90×10^4	4.28
Escherichia coli	Epoxy	10 min	2.07×10^4	5.31
Clostridium sporogenes	Epoxy	10 min	1.83×10^4	1.68

Sodium Hypochlorite at 0.52% in WFI

Organism Tested	Surface	Wetted Period	Initial Positive Control Inoculate	Results in Log Reduction
Candida albicans	Stainless Steel	5 min	1.09×10^4	4.04
Aspergillus brasiliensis	Stainless Steel	5 min	5.00×10^4	4.71
Staphylococcus aureus	Stainless Steel	5 min	2.75×10^3	3.44
Escherichia coli	Stainless Steel	5 min	4.30×10^3	3.63
Pseudomonas aeruginosa	Stainless Steel	5 min	1.55×10^3	3.19
Bacillus subtilis	Stainless Steel	5 min	6.65×10^3	3.82
Penicillium glabrum	Stainless Steel	5 min	4.50×10^3	3.73
Streptomyces flavovirens	Stainless Steel	5 min	2.20×10^4	4.34
Micrococcus luteus	Stainless Steel	5 min	2.33×10^4	4.37
Bacillus infantis	Stainless Steel	5 min	1.44×10^5	3.38
Candida albicans	Stainless Steel	10 min	1.09×10^4	4.04
Aspergillus brasiliensis	Stainless Steel	10 min	5.00×10^4	4.7
Staphylococcus aureus	Stainless Steel	10 min	2.75×10^3	3.44
Escherichia coli	Stainless Steel	10 min	4.30×10^3	3.63
Pseudomonas aeruginosa	Stainless Steel	10 min	1.55×10^3	3.19
Bacillus subtilis	Stainless Steel	10 min	5.30×10^3	3.72

Penicillium glabrum	Stainless Steel	10 min	5.40×10^3	3.73
Streptomyces flavovirens	Stainless Steel	10 min	2.20×10^4	4.34
Micrococcus luteus	Stainless Steel	10 min	2.33×10^4	4.37
Bacillus infantis	Stainless Steel	10 min	1.44×10^5	3.70
Candida albicans	Epoxy	5 min	1.61×10^4	4.21
Aspergillus brasiliensis	Epoxy	5 min	7.95×10^4	4.9
Staphylococcus aureus	Epoxy	5 min	1.10×10^3	3.04
Escherichia coli	Epoxy	5 min	6.20×10^3	3.79
Pseudomonas aeruginosa	Epoxy	5 min	1.65×10^3	3.22
Bacillus subtilis	Epoxy	5 min	6.45×10^3	3.81
Penicillium glabrum	Epoxy	5 min	8.40×10^3	3.92
Streptomyces flavovirens	Epoxy	5 min	2.28×10^4	4.36
Micrococcus luteus	Epoxy	5 min	7.30×10^4	4.86
Bacillus infantis	Epoxy	5 min	1.07×10^4	4.03
Candida albicans	Epoxy	10 min	1.61×10^4	4.21
Aspergillus brasiliensis	Epoxy	10 min	7.95×10^4	4.9
Staphylococcus aureus	Epoxy	10 min	1.10×10^3	3.04
Escherichia coli	Epoxy	10 min	6.20×10^3	3.79
Pseudomonas aeruginosa	Epoxy	10 min	1.65×10^3	3.22
Bacillus subtilis	Epoxy	10 min	6.45×10^3	3.81
Penicillium glabrum	Epoxy	10 min	8.40×10^3	3.92
Streptomyces flavovirens	Epoxy	10 min	2.28×10^4	4.36
Micrococcus luteus	Epoxy	10 min	7.30×10^4	4.86
Bacillus infantis	Epoxy	10 min	1.07×10^4	4.03

Sodium Hypochlorite at 0.25% in WFI

Organism Tested	Surface	Wetted Period	Initial Positive Control Inoculate	Results in Log Reduction
Staphylococcus aureus	Epoxy Floor	5 min	1.89×10^6	4.58
Pseudomonas aeruginosa	Epoxy Floor	5 min	1.69×10^6	4.53
Candida albicans	Epoxy Floor	5 min	2.20×10^6	4.64
Aspergillus brasiliensis	Epoxy Floor	5 min	5.85×10^4	3.07
Penicillium citrinum	Epoxy Floor	5 min	1.40×10^5	3.7
Penicillium glabrum	Epoxy Floor	5 min	1.66×10^5	3.52
Bacillus licheniformis	Epoxy Floor	5 min	4.30×10^4	1.58
Staphylococcus aureus	Epoxy Floor	10 min	1.89×10^6	4.58
Pseudomonas aeruginosa	Epoxy Floor	10 min	1.69×10^6	4.53
Candida albicans	Epoxy Floor	10 min	2.20×10^6	4.64
Aspergillus brasiliensis	Epoxy Floor	10 min	5.85×10^4	3.07
Penicillium citrinum	Epoxy Floor	10 min	1.40×10^5	2.59
Penicillium glabrum	Epoxy Floor	10 min	1.66×10^5	3.52
Bacillus licheniformis	Epoxy Floor	10 min	4.30×10^4	2.37

Staphylococcus aureus	Vinyl Floor	5 min	2.00×10^6	4.60
Pseudomonas aeruginosa	Vinyl Floor	5 min	4.93×10^6	4.99
Candida albicans	Vinyl Floor	5 min	1.87×10^6	4.57
Aspergillus brasiliensis	Vinyl Floor	5 min	7.15×10^4	3.15
Penicillium citrinum	Vinyl Floor	5 min	1.48×10^5	3.47
Penicillium glabrum	Vinyl Floor	5 min	1.89×10^5	3.58
Bacillus licheniformis	Vinyl Floor	5 min	5.10×10^4	2.07
Staphylococcus aureus	Vinyl Floor	10 min	2.00×10^6	4.60
Pseudomonas aeruginosa	Vinyl Floor	10 min	4.93×10^6	4.99
Candida albicans	Vinyl Floor	10 min	1.87×10^6	4.57
Aspergillus brasiliensis	Vinyl Floor	10 min	7.15×10^4	3.15
Penicillium citrinum	Vinyl Floor	10 min	1.48×10^5	3.47
Penicillium glabrum	Vinyl Floor	10 min	1.89×10^5	3.58
Bacillus licheniformis	Vinyl Floor	10 min	5.10×10^4	3.19

Hydrogen Peroxide at 6% in WFI

Organism Tested	Surface	Wetted Period	Initial Positive Control Inoculate	Results in Log Reduction
Staphylococcus aureus	Stainless Steel	5 min	9.00×10^3	1.85
Pseudomonas aeruginosa	Stainless Steel	5 min	3.50×10^3	2.14
Candida albicans	Stainless Steel	5 min	2.00×10^5	0.91
Cladosporium cladosporiodes	Stainless Steel	5 min	1.70×10^4	0.53
Staphylococcus aureus	Glass	5 min	6.00×10^3	2.89
Pseudomonas aeruginosa	Glass	5 min	8.50×10^2	2.93
Candida albicans	Glass	5 min	2.15×10^5	1.36
Cladosporium cladosporiodes	Glass	5 min	1.65×10^4	1.3

3.12 RESISTANCE THEORIES TO GERMICIDAL AGENTS

In present times, resistance to antibiotics by certain organisms in the human body has become more than a theory. Recent publications have even shown the possible presence of "superbugs" that have become immune to certain antibiotics and require new interventions. The human body has a very complex internal system whereby mainly blood makeup and circulation, tissue, and absorption make it very difficult to assure that a drug product is adequately delivered to the specific location where an infection is noted in the concentration required to destroy the contaminate in question. At the same time the level or dose of antimicrobial agent (an antibiotic and an example) is minimal as reactions, toxicity, and adverse effects of too strong a drug product may cause a multitude of complications within the human body that can range from simple rashes to liver and kidney complications.

With the initial fever surrounding resistance in the human body many scientists in the pharmaceutical and biotechnology world began to ponder a theory of whether such resistance could occur between biocidal agents and organisms vested in the clean room environment. However, such complexity does not occur between biocidal agents and microorganisms. Within the clean room environment hard surfaces that may or may not have porosity are the "patient to be treated" Only surfaces can be disinfected with biocidal agents. Air within the clean room cannot be disinfected to any feasible degree, only filtered. On a surface, very little blocks the disinfectant from contacting the contamination. To a small degree, organisms may vest themselves in pores of the substrate and at the same time soil load or residual can block the biocidal agent from contacting the organism. While porosity of the surface and soil load are a concern, they are not an equivalent to the concerns that exist within the human body. Antimicrobial effectiveness of biocidal agents does not resemble at all that of human products. The simplicity of the surface to be disinfected and the ability to use biocidal agents of enormously high strength increase the disinfectants ability to destroy microorganisms far beyond that of an antibiotic.

Studies performed and published by this author showed that organisms subjected to antimicrobial effectiveness testing and surviving organisms regrown and retested showed that resistance was unfounded (see "Assessing Resistance and Appropriate Acceptance Criteria of Biocidal Agents" in References section). Simply said, after conducting studies for five years on over 70 organisms, resistance was not found to exist. This theory, supported by the Parenteral Drug Association, PDA Technical Report #70 is just that: an unproven theory.

3.13 CONCLUSION

Unfortunately, antimicrobial agents are not the single means to attain an acceptable environment. There is no magic chemical that when used suddenly creates the perfect environment. Many integral factors in a wholistic approach combine to create a successful system. Control of the environment is one of the keys to success. Antimicrobial agents are the corrective action for a poor control system. This being said, they are an imperfect solution and provide no preventative assurances after they have dried. Understanding the entire contamination control spectrum is the key to success. Often in the good manufacturing practice world we just invoke a few levels of a complete contamination control system and by doing so find ourselves with contamination excursions. The successful contamination control professional takes into account all aspects required for a complete system and assures that all aspects are implemented, tested, documented and include the appropriate training and retraining of personnel. Only a complete system assures success and routine, repeatable success.

3.14 SPECIAL ACKNOWLEDGMENT

A special Thank you to Kelly Rocco, Manager QA, Veltek Associates, Inc. for collecting and reporting VAI Laboratory Antimicrobial Efficacy Performance Testing Summaries.

BIBLIOGRAPHY

1. Block, Seymour Stanton (ed.), *Disinfection, Sterilization and Preservation,* 4th Edition. Philadelphia, PA: Lea and Febiger, 1991
2. McDonnell, Gerald and A. Denver Russell, Antiseptics and Disinfectants: Activity, Action, and Resistance, *Clinical Microbiological Reviews,* Jan 1999.
3. Vellutato, Arthur, L. Jr. Assessing Resistance and Appropriate Acceptance Criteria of Biocidal Agents. In *Contamination Control in Healthcare Products Manufacturing,* edited by Russell Madsen and Jeanne Moldenhauer, DHI, LLC, Chapter 9, Pages 319–352, 2014.
4. Vellutato, Arthur, L. Jr., Implementing a Cleaning and Disinfection Program in Pharmaceutical and Biotechnology Clean Room Environments. In *Laboratory Validation: A Practitioner's Guide,* edited by Jeanne Moldenhauer, DHI, LLC, Chapter 8, Pages 179–230, 2003.
5. Aseptic Processing, Inc. (API) a division of Veltek Associates, Inc., Validation and Testing Studies Surrounding the Resistance of Biocidal Agents, 2009.
6. Center for Drugs and Biologics and Office of Regulatory Affairs, Food and Drug Administration, Guidelines on Sterile Drug Products produced by Aseptic Processing, p. 9, June 1987.
7. Center for Drugs and Biologics and Office of Regulatory Affairs, Food and Drug Administration, Sterile Drug Products Produced by Aseptic Processing Draft, Concept paper (Not for Implementation), September 27, 2002.
8. EU GMP Annex 1: Manufacture of Sterile Medicinal Products, November 25, 2008 (rev).
9. AOAC International, *Official Methods of Analysis,* 16th Ed., 5th Revision. Gaithersburg, MD: AOAC, 1998.
10. Parenteral Drug Association (PDA), Technical Report #70 (TR70). Bethesda, MD: PDA, 2015.
11. European Committee for Standardization, Chemical Disinfectants and Antiseptics – Quantitative non-porous surface test for the evaluation of bactericidal and/or fungicidal activity of chemical disinfectants used in food, industrial, domestic and institutional areas –Test methods and requirements without mechanical action (phase 2/step2), EN 13697 E, ICS 11.080.20; 71.100.35. Brussels, 2001.
12. FB Engineering, Efficacy Testing of Biocidal Products – Overview of Available Tests. At the request of the Swedish Chemicals Agency. Table 1, pages 24–189, 2008.
13. Australian Government Department of Health and Aging, Therapeutics Goods Administration (TGA) Guidelines for the Evaluation of Sterilants and Disinfectants, February 1998.
14. Connor, D. E. and M. K. Eckman, Rotation of Phenolic Disinfectants, *Pharmaceutical Technology,* 148–158, September 1992.
15. Vellutato, Arthur, Sr., United States Patent 6,123,900. United States Patent Office, 1992.
16. Vellutato, Arthur, Jr., Validation of the Core2Clean Spray Mop Fog Systems, Internal Validation Report, Veltek Associates, Inc. January 2000.

4 The Microbiome and Its Usefulness to Decontamination/ Disinfection Practices

Jeanne Moldenhauer

CONTENTS

4.1 WHAT IS THE HUMAN MICROBIOME?

Within the human body there are both human cells and microorganisms present. They work together to perform the necessary functions of the body. Collectively, these organisms, cells, and environmental interactions are called the human microbiome (Wilder et al., 2013).

The complexity of the ecosystem within the body affects many different bodily functions, e.g., digestion, immunity, resistance to pathogens, and many more. The information that can be gained by understanding the human microbiome can significantly enhance our knowledge of the human body (Wilder et al., 2013).

4.2 INTRODUCTION – THE HUMAN MICROBIOME PROJECT (HMP)

The United States National Institutes of Health (NIH) launched an initiative in 2008 to identify and characterize the microorganisms that are found in both healthy and diseased individuals. This initiative is called the Human Microbiome Project (HMP). It was believed that this project would take about five years to complete, with a budget of $115 million (Wikipedia, 2018).

There were many goals established as part of this program including (Wikipedia, 2018):

- Use of methods that did not require media or culturing to characterize the microorganisms. One of these types of methods is metagenomics. Metagenomics is the study of genomes that are recovered from environmental samples. It is the differentiation of genomes from multiple organisms or individuals. The organisms may be either in a symbiotic relationship, or at a crime scene.
- It was also deemed important to provide a genetic sequence of the entire genome.
- An emphasis was defined on five areas of the human body: oral, skin, vaginal, gut, and nasal/lung microbiology. Funding was provided to perform 16 s rRNA sequencing using polymerase chain reaction from humans. 16 s rRNA sequencing is the part of the 30 S small subunit of a prokaryotic ribosome, which binds to the Shine-Dalgarno sequence. The genes coding for this part of the genome are often used in constructing phylogenies because this area has a slow rate of evolution in this part of the gene.
- Development of a reference set of the microbial genomic sequences, and preliminary characterizing of the human microbiome.
- Exploration of the relationship between disease and changes in the human microbiome.
- Generation of new technologies and/or tools to perform the necessary computational analysis.
- Establishment of a resource repository.
- Evaluation of the impacts of the ethical, legal, and social implications regarding the human microbiome research.

4.3   TESTING AND RESULTS OF THE HUMAN MICROBIOME PROJECT

Scientific journals and reports since 2014 have indicated a high number of microorganisms living in the human body. Some actually claim that there are ten times the number of microbial cells versus those of bacteria (American Academy of Microbiology, 2014; Rosner, 2014). Rosner (2014) also identifies that this number may be highly variable, due to the nutritional condition of the individual, body size, age, ethnicity, culture, and environment. It was further postulated that the variability is affected by the diversity of humans, the diversity of environments, and effects due to the stage of life. Based upon these factors, there is a high level of variability in these relationships between human and microbial cells. Additionally, there is variability in the number of cells present in the human body. One report (American Academy of Microbiology, 2014) estimated that the human body contains approximately 37 trillion cells. In this case, the relationship of microbial cells to human cells is about 3:1.

Additional reports were published in 2016 with different estimates of the relationships between human and microbial cells. Sender et al. (2016) provided estimates of the relationship being 1:1. It was estimated that the uncertainty is about 25% and the variation approximately 53% (Sender et al., 2016; Abbott, 2016).

It is important to note that many of the organisms comprising the human microbiome have not been cultured or characterized completely. Generally, they are considered to be bacteria, single-cell eukaryotes, helminth parasites, viruses and bacteriophages (viruses of bacteria) (Wikipedia, 2018).

4.3.1 WORK COMPLETED FOR THE HUMAN MICROBIOME PROJECT

This project resulted in numerous peer-reviewed publications that were sponsored by the Human Microbiome Project (NIH, 2018). The following identifies some of the various work that was funded as part of the Human Microbiome Project (NIH, 2018; Wikipedia, 2018):

- Creation of a massive database to organize, store, access, search, and annotate the data generated, including: The Integrated Microbial Genomes (database and analysis system), a related system for metagenome data sets, the CharProDB database of characterized protein annotations, and the Genomes on Line Database (GOLD). The GOLD database monitors the status of genomic and metagenomic projects and data worldwide.
- Developing tools for comparative analysis of patterns, themes, and trends in complex data sets. For example: The RAPSearch2 (a protein similarity tool), Boulder Alignment Editor (ALE) for web-based RNA alignment, WebMGA for fast metagenomic sequence analysis, and DNACLUST for accurate and efficient clustering of phylogenetic markers.
- Developing new methods and system for assembly of massive data sets of sequences. This required development of new algorithms.
- Creation of a catalog of sequenced reference genomes of pure bacterial strains from different body sites.
- Creation of a central repository of all Human Microbiome Project data.
- Conduct of studies to evaluate the legal and ethical issues surrounding the whole genome sequencing research.
- New methods to predict the active transcription factor binding sites.
- Identification of a widely distributed ribosomally produced electron carrier precursor.
- Creation of time-lapse moving pictures of the human microbiome.
- Found a dominant role played by *Verrucomicrobia* in soil bacterial communities, that was previously unknown.
- Found factors that determined the virulence potential of *Garnerella vaginalis* strains in vaginosis.
- Found a link between oral microbiota and atherosclerosis.
- Found factors distinguishing the microbiota of healthy and diseased gut.
- In 2012, a database was established including the normal microbial makeup of healthy individuals using genome sequencing techniques and normal variations.

- Found that the microorganisms present provide more genes responsible for human survival that the humans' own genes.
- Found that certain metabolic activities like the digestion of fats are not always conducted by the same bacterial species.
- And many more findings.

4.4 APPLICATIONS OF THE HUMAN MICROBIOME PROJECT TO REGULATED INDUSTRIES

The information generated from the human microbiome project has a significant impact on pharmaceutical microbiology. This includes the development, production, and use of therapeutic products along with the controlled environments where medicinal products are produced (Wilder et al., 2013).

Wilder et al. (2013) identified potential ways that the Human Microbiome Project may affect pharmaceutical microbiology. One example included: the use of antimicrobial preserved products being introduced to humans may be compromised depending upon the variation in the microbiome and potentially result in overgrowth of the pathogen. They also indicated that the microbiome could influence the response to pharmaceutical products.

4.4.1 Applicable Regulatory Requirements

There are some references in the *Code of Federal Regulations* Title 21 (FDA, 2018):

- 21 CFR 211.84(d)(6) – "Each lot of a component, drug product container, or closure with potential for microbiological contamination that is objectionable in view of its intended use shall be subjected to microbiological tests before use."
- 21 CFR 211.113(a) – "Appropriate written procedures, designed to prevent objectionable microorganisms in drug products not required to be sterile, shall be established and followed."
- 21 CFR 211.165(b) – "There shall be appropriate laboratory testing, as necessary, of each batch of drug product required to be free of objectionable microorganisms."

While these regulatory citations refer to objectionable microorganisms, there is not a single listing of what those organisms are. The affected microorganisms are based upon the intended use of the product, the risk of the microorganism to the patient population, the patient's health, dosage, and frequency of use. For sterile medications, the presence of any microorganisms in the finished product is considered objectionable, regardless of the organism or its concentration. Non-sterile medicines are more difficult, as one expects some contamination to be present. The more that is known about those organisms that are part of the microbiome, the more we can learn about the potential for contamination in our facilities and products (Wilder et al., 2013).

To best use all of this information, it becomes important for the pharmaceutical company to utilize a good system for microbial characterization and identification. Depending upon the regulated industry of use, this may be a phenotypic method or a genomic method. Many companies today have found it useful to utilize a proteonomic system (e.g., Maldi-TOF) due to its accuracy, high throughput, and low cost of use.

Some considerations for a good microbial identification include (Wilder et al, 2013):

- The type of product: What type of product is it? Is it growth-promoting? Is it preserved? Is it an aqueous-based product?
- What is the potential of the microorganism to survive in the product for long periods of time? Are there sufficient nutrients available? Is it the right environment for microbial growth?
- The type of microorganism: Is it a pathogen? Will it cause problems for the patient? If present, can the organism be detected?
- How many microorganisms are recovered?
- Is the microorganism capable of releasing microbial toxins? Could these toxins cause a problem for the patient?
- How is the product administered?
- Who will be getting the medication? Are the patients immune-compromised? Are other diseases an issue?
- What other medications are used by the patient? Is there a likelihood of drug interactions?

All of these considerations should be subjected to risk analysis to determine whether any patient threats exist (Wilder et al., 2013).

4.4.2   USES OF THE HUMAN MICROBIOME PROJECT FOR DECONTAMINATION AND DISINFECTION PROCEDURES

As data is gathered and reviewed for the types of microorganisms present in the human body, this information can be reviewed for its impact on decontamination and disinfection procedures. For example, when these organisms are completely characterized, information may be available to show sensitivities or resistances to various antimicrobial agents, e.g., *mec* genes. As we understand the likelihood of human contamination with specific organisms and the potential for difficulties in eliminating these organisms we will be able to significantly improve our decontamination and disinfection procedures.

We also may be able to develop proactive methods to prevent contamination with some of these microorganisms. Another concern is whether the contamination found at a site really is a human-borne organism. Many investigations start out with typical wording that the contaminant is a human-borne organism. Rarely do we really find if the contaminant was sourced from our operators, or whether it was present on the materials or surfaces in the room. We may find that other items were really the source of contamination in the area, and provide us with greater understanding of our processes and procedures.

LITERATURE CITED

Abbott, A. (2016) Scientists bust myth that our bodies have more bacteria than human cells. *Nature News*. Downloaded from: www.nature.com/news/scientists-bust-myth-that-our-bodies-have-more-bacteria-than-human-cells-1.19136 on January 31, 2018.

American Academy of Microbiology (2014) FAQ: Human Microbiome. Downloaded from: www.asm.org/index.php/aamindex.php/faq-series/5122-humanmicrobiome on January 31, 2018.

Food and Drugs Administration (FDA) (2018) *Code of Federal Regulations Title 21*. 21 CFR 211.84(d)(6) 21 CFR 211.113(a) and 21 CFR 211.165(b).

National Institutes of Health (NIH) (2018) Publications. Human Microbiome Project. Downloaded from: www.hmpdacc.org/hmp/publications.php on January 31, 2018.

Rosner, J. K. (2014) Ten Times More Microbial Cells than Body Cells in Humans? *Microbe Magazine* (February 2014). Downloaded from: www.asmscience.org/content/journal/microbe/10.1128/microbe.9.47.2 on January 31, 2018.

Sender, R., Fuchs, S., and Milo, R. (2016) Are We Really Vastly Outnumbered? Revisiting the Ration of Bacterial to Host Cells in Humans. *Cell* 164(3): 337–340.

Wikipedia (2018) The Human Microbiome Project. Downloaded from: https://en.wikipedia.org/wiki/Human_Microbiome_Project on January 30, 2018.

Wilder, C., Sandle, T., and Sutton, S. (2013) Implications of the Human Microbiome on Pharmaceutical Microbiology. *American Pharmaceutical Review On-Line*. Downloaded from: www.americanpharmaceuticalreview.com/1504-White-Papers-Application-Notes/140112-Implications-of-the-Human-Microbiome-on-Pharmaceutical-Microbiology/ on January 20, 2018.

5 Disinfectant Qualification Testing Considerations for Critical Manufacturing Environments

Dave Rottjakob and Christine Chan

CONTENTS

5.1 INTRODUCTION

Obtaining the highest confidence that critical manufacturing environments are properly cleaned, sanitized and disinfected is paramount in ensuring the production of safe pharmaceutical products and medical devices. The microbiological risk of these products is primarily determined by the quality of raw materials, the integrity of the manufacturing process, and the effectiveness of cleaning and disinfection procedures performed in the facility. It is for this reason that the U.S. Food and Drug

Administration (FDA) requires the manufacturers of these products and devices to qualify and validate the disinfection procedures used in the aseptic, cleanroom, and other critical production environments. This chapter provides an overview of disinfection qualification testing and the considerations that must be addressed when designing and executing these studies.

5.2   THE IMPORTANCE OF DISINFECTION QUALIFICATION STUDIES

Disinfection qualifications effectively mitigate the microbial contamination that may occur during the manufacture of a product. Mitigating the risk of contamination ultimately helps to ensure a safe product for the end-user or patient. Control of microbial contamination is required by the FDA's Current Good Manufacturing Practice for Finished Pharmaceuticals as defined in 21 CFR §211.113 which states the following requirements:

5.2.1   CONTROL OF MICROBIOLOGICAL CONTAMINATION

a. Appropriate written procedures, designed to prevent objectionable microorganisms in drug products not required to be sterile, shall be established and followed.
b. Appropriate written procedures, designed to prevent microbiological contamination of drug products purporting to be sterile, shall be established and followed. Such procedures shall include validation of all aseptic and sterilization processes.

These requirements are additionally clarified in the FDA's 2004 Guidance for Industry, "Drug Products Produced by Processing – Current Good Manufacturing Practice." This guidance also addresses disinfection qualification.

5.2.2   DISINFECTION EFFICACY

The suitability, efficacy, and limitations of disinfecting agents and procedures should be assessed. The effectiveness of these disinfectants and procedures should be measured by their ability to ensure that potential contaminants are adequately removed from surfaces.

While federal regulations and guidance documents mandate microbial control of sterile and non-sterile manufacturing environments, the interpretation and enforcement of these regulations can be seen through good manufacturing practice (GMP) inspections and the resulting FDA Form 483 warning letters. The extent of the deficiencies listed in a FDA-483 warning letter can mean the difference between being operational or being shut down. It has been well documented that the observations citing "the failure to ensure disinfection" in 483 warning letters have been trending upward.

5.2.3   EXCERPTS FROM FDA FORM 483 WARNING LETTERS

"Your disinfectant qualification for (b)(4) and (b)(4) bi-spore disinfectants documented that the log reduction criteria (Bacteria>4, Fungi>3) was not met when challenged with multiple organisms in a variety of surfaces. After disinfection, you recovered *Micrococcus luteus* on vinyl, (b)(4), stainless steel, glass and wall laminate and *Enterobacter cloacae, Rhodococcus* sp, *Burkholderia cepacia, Pseudomonas aeruginosa, Methylobacterium mesophilicum* and, *Acinetobacter lwoffi* on glass. However your procedures for routine cleaning of the aseptic manufacturing area continue to require the use of unqualified disinfectants during days (b)(4) through (b)(4) of your disinfection program." Warning letter dated October 7, 2011.

"The qualification of your disinfectant (b)(4) failed to demonstrate that it is suitable and effective to remove microorganisms from different surfaces. Specifically, this disinfectant failed to meet the qualification criteria when challenged with multiple organisms." Warning letter dated October 7, 2011.

"The coupons used in the 'Disinfectant Efficacy Verification for Hard Surfaces' VP-2008-065-PV approved: 04/26/2010, were not representative of the surfaces found in the XXX laboratories. For example, (b)(4) was used in the study to represent the biological safety cabinets, laminar flow hoods, and tables in the processing and manufacturing areas. However, the equipment is comprised of (b)(4)." Warning letter dated January 29, 2013.

"Your firm failed to establish and follow appropriate written procedures that are designed to prevent microbiological contamination of drug products purporting to be sterile, and that include validation of all aseptic and sterilization processes (21 CFR 211.113(b))." Warning letter dated April 22, 2014.

"Your firm failed to ensure the system for cleaning and disinfecting equipment is adequate to produce aseptic conditions. (21 CFR 211.42(c)(10)(v))." Warning letter dated May 5, 2016.

"We observed that your firm did not adequately disinfect your RABS. For example, surfaces (b)(4) the RABS (b)(4) were not routinely disinfected, and your firm incompletely disinfected the bottom of the RABS (b)(4). In addition, you have not sufficiently established the efficacy of disinfectants you use in aseptic processing cleanrooms. Your disinfectant study only challenged (b)(4) and (b)(4) manufacturing surfaces. You did not provide an adequate scientific rationale for not challenging other representative surfaces, such as glass windows, (b)(4), (b)(4), (b)(4), (b)(4), or other interior RABS surfaces. In response to this letter, provide data to support the efficacy of your disinfection procedures on additional representative surfaces." Warning letter dated November 16, 2016.

"Our inspection found multiple deficient practices at your facility that pose a significant microbiological contamination risk. For example, your cleaning and disinfection program lacked use of a sporicidal agent. Significantly, the microbe identified in the sterility failures is a spore-former. In addition, our inspection identified poor facility maintenance. This included leaking pipes in the cleanroom ceiling, chipped and cracked floors in the batch tank room, and blue and black particulates as well as dust on tanks next to the ingredient charging ports.

We acknowledge your commitment to improve your cleaning and sanitization program, including the addition of sporicidal agents to the program. However, a sound disinfectant program also includes a written schedule, sound methods, efficacy studies, and environmental data to support the ongoing effectiveness of the agents." Warning letter dated December 23, 2016.

"Your response stated that you use (b)(4) as your sporicidal agent to disinfect the aseptic processing areas. However, you did not provide supporting documentation for our review, such as the concentration of (b)(4) used and the contact time applied to ensure adequate levels of disinfection." Warning letter dated March 28, 2017.

Resource: www.fda.gov/iceci/enforcementactions/WarningLetters/default.htm

5.3   DIFFERENCE BETWEEN DISINFECTION QUALIFICATION AND VALIDATION

Disinfection and sanitization in pharmaceutical and other controlled manufacturing spaces refers to the killing, inactivation, removal, or reduction of contaminating microorganisms to levels considered safe per industry standards and regulations. The terms "cleanroom disinfection qualification," "disinfection validation," and "cleaning validation" are often used in the pharmaceutical and aseptic manufacturing industries interchangeably. While these terms seem to define the same thing, they actually are rather different. In fact, validations build upon qualifications.

5.3.1   DISINFECTION QUALIFICATION

Formally evaluating the efficacy and suitability of antimicrobial products and procedures used to eliminate contaminant microorganisms on various surface types and components within an aseptic, sterile, or otherwise controlled manufacturing environment. Disinfection qualifications are critical in assuring the microbial control of a manufacturing environment by qualifying the appropriate use and effectiveness of disinfection products and procedures.

5.3.2   DISINFECTION VALIDATION

Validating that sterile, aseptic, and even non-sterile manufacturing environments are under microbial control as measured by a comprehensive and continuous environmental monitoring program.

5.3.3   CLEANING VALIDATION

Studies designed to measure a procedure's effectiveness at removing by-products or residual chemicals which may result during the manufacturing process.

5.4   THE FDA REQUIRES DISINFECTION QUALIFICATION STUDIES

United States Pharmacopoeia (USP) <1072> "Disinfectants and Antiseptics" clarifies that a Disinfection Qualification study "is considered necessary since critical process steps like disinfection of aseptic processing areas, as required by GMP regulation, need to be validated and the EPA registration requirements do not address how disinfectants are used in the pharmaceutical, biotechnological and medical device industries."

Before disinfectant products can be sold in the United States, the products must be "registered" with the Environmental Protection Agency (EPA) to support the efficacy label claims. To generate disinfection claims, standardized testing is performed using quality control strain microorganisms (e.g., *Staphylococcus aureus* and *Pseudomonas aeruginosa*) on a single representative hard surface such as stainless steel or glass. In contrast to these claims, the manufacturing environment utilizes a variety of surface types and encounters a variety of environmental microbes.

A disinfectant product that has a standard label claim for efficacy on stainless steel or glass surfaces often does not demonstrate the same level of efficacy on other surface types against the specific environmental isolates found in the manufacturing environment. Therefore, disinfection assessment techniques must be modified to evaluate the true uses of the product in these environments. Another typical example of the importance of assessment technique is to increase the contact time from what is listed on the disinfectant product label to achieve the desired efficacy.

Table 5.1 displays an example of the differences that may be found in $\log_{10}$ reductions using the same test organism and disinfectant on multiple surface types. The table illustrates that with the particular disinfectant studied, microbial reduction from plastic surfaces was relatively less efficient than from stainless steel surface. The anomalies are highlighted below.

5.4.1 When to Conduct Disinfection Qualification Studies

The ideal time in the product development lifecycle to conduct a disinfection qualification study is during the construction of the manufacturing facility. This time frame puts the study before operation of the facility when disinfection processes and products are being considered. The latest a qualification should be performed is before

---

TABLE 5.1

Example Results from Efficacy of a Cleaning Product on Microorganism Reduction on Multiple Surface Types

Active Ingredient (5 min. Exposure Time)	$\log_{10}$ Reduction of Environmental Isolate (*Staphylococcus* sp.) on the Following Routine Surfaces							
	PVC	Lexan	Vinyl	Epoxy	Stainless Steel	Polypropylene	Glass	Polyethylene
Peracetic acid/ Hydrogen peroxide	>4.56	>4.39	>4.48	>4.33	>4.74	>4.19	>4.57	>4.31
Quaternary Ammonium	>4.03	>4.10	**2.78**	4.19	>4.04	**2.62**	>4.35	>4.60
Hydrogen Peroxide	**1.58**	**1.23**	**<1.27**	**1.79**	>3.79	**<0.85**	**1.68**	**1.33**
Sodium Hypochlorite	>4.25	>4.18	>4.77	>4.19	>3.95	3.88	>4.09	>4.31
Alkaline Phenolic	>4.03	>4.39	**2.65**	4.28	>4.94	**<1.02**	>5.25	**1.68**

starting a full scale GMP manufacturing operation and before an FDA GMP audit. Unfortunately, disinfection qualifications are often performed reactively instead of proactively, in response to a product contamination, an environmental monitoring excursion, or to the observations listed in the FDA Form 483 warning letter. Waiting to perform a qualification study in these scenarios can lead to a cease in manufacturing operations and the commissioning of a disinfection qualification studies that go well beyond the need of the operation.

Once the procedures have been qualified, the manufacturing environment should be continuously monitored to identify newly trending environmental isolates. This allows manufacturing facilities to successfully determine when additional disinfection qualification testing is necessary. In addition, supplemental qualifications should be performed following a change in a disinfectant product, a modification in cleaning or disinfection procedures, and the incorporation of new surfaces into the cleanroom or aseptic manufacturing area.

5.5 DECIDING HOW TO PERFORM DISINFECTION QUALIFICATION STUDIES

Unfortunately, there is no standard method outlining step-by-step instructions of *how* disinfection qualifications studies should be conducted. However, general guidance can be found in the United States Pharmacopeia (USP) <1072> document and in the American Society for Testing and Materials (ASTM) International E2614 guidance document. The following is a summary of that guidance:

5.5.1 SUSPENSION-BASED TESTING VERSUS COUPON-BASED TESTING

In general, disinfectant efficacy evaluations are made using either suspension-based methods or coupon/surface-based methods. Suspension methods evaluate the reduction of a known organism population inoculated directly into a sample of the liquid disinfectant. Following inoculation and the observation of a predetermined contact time, samples of the inoculated substance are removed, neutralized and evaluated for survivors as compared to an untreated control suspension. Since the simulation of organism films on the specific environmental surface types are not accounted for in this method, it is recommended that suspension-based tests be used only for initial disinfectant screening purposes.

In contrast, coupon/surface-based testing is more rigorous and involves the formation of a dried organism film onto representative surface types that best simulates the contaminated environment. The surfaces are then exposed with the disinfectant utilizing a simulated-use procedure. Following a predetermined contact time, each surface is neutralized and surviving organisms are enumerated in a quantitative fashion for comparison to untreated surfaces.

As is evidenced by FDA 483 warning letters, coupon-based testing is ultimately required to qualify disinfectants used in the pharmaceutical and aseptic manufacturing arena.

5.5.2 Scope of Qualification Testing

Each manufacturing facility is different; therefore, each qualification study is different. Considering the various combinations of surfaces, organisms, disinfectant products and disinfection procedures, these studies can become rather complex. Tables 5.2, 5.3, and 5.4 list common considerations that contribute to the complexity of these tests and help illustrate why careful scientific rationale should be used in the design of the studies.

In addition to the aforementioned testing considerations, the following technical elements, among others, must be given serious consideration while developing the scope of the study:

- Coupon/carrier preparation
- Organism preparation, and coupon inoculation
- Drying conditions for optimal organism viability
- Disinfectant preparation
- Determination and testing of expiration time for diluted or activated products
- Disinfectant application and exposure times
- Neutralization of coupons and recovery of survivors
- Disinfectant performance criteria (e.g., contact time and concentration)

The explanation of these technical elements falls outside of the scope of this document and is best suited to a future chapter.

The following section provides an overview of the procedures commonly used in these studies:

TABLE 5.2
Surface Types

Surface Types Commonly Found in the
Pharmaceutical/Aseptic Manufacturing Environment

Stainless steel (304 or 316 grade)

Polyvinyl chloride (PVC)

Glass

Lexan® (plexiglass)

Polyethylene

Tyvek

Terazzo tile

Teflon

Polypropylene

Fiberglass-reinforced Plastic

Anodized aluminum alloys

TABLE 5.3

Challenge Microorganisms

Typical Challenge Microorganisms Used in Disinfection
Qualification Studies

Standard Reference Isolates	Environmental Isolates
Vegetative Bacteria	
Staphylococcus aureus	*Micrococcus luteus*
Escherichia coli	*Staphylococcus hominis*
Pseudomonas aeruginosa	*Staphylococcus epidermidis*
	Burkholderia cepacia
	Corynebacterium species
Yeast and Mold (Fungi)	
Candida albicans	*Aspergillus* species
Aspergillus brasiliensis	*Penicillium* species
Penicillium chrysogenum	
Spore-forming Bacteria	
Bacillus subtilis	*Bacillus* species
	Paenibacillus glucanolyticus

TABLE 5.4

Typical Active Ingredients and Typical Method Applications

Active Ingredients of Typical Disinfectant Products Used in Aseptic Manufacturing	Typical Methods for Application of Disinfectants in the Aseptic Manufacturing Environment
Peracetic acid/Hydrogen Peroxide	Mop-on
Quaternary Ammonium	Spray
Alcohol (Ethanol/Isopropyl)	Wipe
Sodium Hypochlorite	Flood
Alkaline Phenolic	With or without rinse step
Acidic Phenolic	With or without squeegee
Hydrogen Peroxide	Fogging or submersion

5.6   OVERVIEW OF STUDY DESIGN

Once study parameters have been established, a testing protocol is developed. The overall testing process is generally executed as follows. Each surface coupon is individually inoculated with the test organism. A sufficient number of coupons must be inoculated to evaluate each disinfectant, each test organism and each disinfection procedure for each coupon replicate. The coupons are placed into an incubator to allow the test organism to dry as a film. Once dried, each coupon is treated and exposed to the disinfectant. Following careful monitoring of the exposure, each coupon is transferred to a preselected solution designed to neutralize the disinfectant and suspend or rinse off any surviving test organisms. This solution is quantitatively evaluated to enumerate the number of survivors onto an appropriate agar plate medium. Inoculated, but untreated (not exposed to disinfectant) control coupons are similarly enumerated to determine the initial level of test organism on each surface type prior to treatment. Appropriate controls should be included with the study to assess the sterility of the materials used in testing and to confirm the adequacy of the neutralization techniques used.

After incubation, the recovery plates are enumerated, and the study controls are evaluated to ensure study validity. Survivors found on the treated coupons are compared to survivors recovered on the untreated control coupons to determine the $\log_{10}$ reductions. The level of reduction observed can then be used to determine the success of the disinfection procedure.

5.7 CONCLUSION

Properly designed, appropriately qualified and consistently executed disinfection procedures are critical to the production of safe and effective pharmaceuticals, medical devices, and other sterile or non-sterile products. As demonstrated in various FDA Form 483 warning letters, the proper qualification of these disinfection procedures is, in fact, a requirement. The major considerations and potential variables that must be addressed when considering the design and execution of a successful disinfection qualification study have been outlined in this document. Careful review of the data collected in properly executed qualification studies will help facilities monitor potential deficiencies in their cleaning and disinfection program. As a result of the disinfection qualification studies, future trends that fall outside the pre-established disinfection program will allow facility staff to investigate and take appropriate corrective action. Furthermore, allowing the facility to re-establish environmental control ultimately ensures a safer product for the end-user or patient.

5.8 ABOUT THE AUTHORS

Dave Rottjakob is the Director of Business Development at Accuratus Lab Services, a contract testing laboratory specializing in disinfection efficacy for the pharmaceutical, medical device, and healthcare, and antimicrobial industries. Rottjakob has more than 20 years' experience in the clinical microbiology, industrial microbiology, and antimicrobial testing industries. His experience ranges from serving as a bench-level clinical laboratory microbiologist to numerous supervisory positions with an established GMP manufacturer of a personal care product, as well as several technical and business development management positions with ATS Labs. Rottjakob has recently served as the secretary of the AOAC International's Methods Committee M on Antimicrobial Efficacy Testing. He has also sat on antimicrobial expert review panels (ERP) for U.S. EPA. Rottjakob earned his Bachelor of Arts degree in biology from St. Mary's University and his Medical Technology/Clinical Laboratory Science degree from St. Paul Ramsey Medical Center. Rottjakob has co-authored of several peer-reviewed studies, publication articles, and white papers, and is a board registered Medical Technologist and Clinical Laboratory Scientist.

Christine Chan is the Technical Sales Manager at Accuratus Lab Services, a contract testing laboratory specializing in disinfection efficacy for the pharmaceutical, medical device, healthcare, and antimicrobial industries. Chan has more than ten years' experience in microbiology, medical device, and genetics/cell biology testing industries. Her experience ranges from bench-level laboratory cell biologist and microbiologist at a genetics research laboratory and at a start-up medical device company, as well as navigating through several technical and business development positions with ATS Labs/Accuratus Lab Services. Chan is an active member of the Parenteral Drug Association Midwest Chapter. Chan has a degree in Genetics, Cell Biology and Development from the University of Minnesota.

REFERENCES

American Society for Testing and Materials (ASTM). Test Method, Standard Guide for Evaluation of Cleanroom Disinfectants, E2614–08.

Block, S. S., *Disinfection, Sterilization, and Preservation*. Lippincott, Williams and Wilkins, Philadelphia, PA, 2001.

Current Good Manufacturing Practice for Finished Pharmaceuticals, 21 CFR Part 211.

Food and Drugs Administration, Inspections, Compliance, Enforcement, and Criminal Investigations. Retrieved www.fda.gov/iceci/enforcementactions/WarningLetters/default.htm, 2013.

Madsen, R. E. and Moldenhauer, J. *Contamination Control in Healthcare Product Manufacturing*, Volume 1, DHI Publishing, River Grove, IL, 2013.

United States Pharmacopeia (USP) 34, Chapter <1072> Disinfection and Antiseptics – General Information, pp.579–580, May 1, 2011.

U.S. Food and Drug Administration (FDA), Guidance for Industry Sterile Drug Products Produced by Aseptic Processing – Current Good Manufacturing Practice, 2004.

6 Methods for Contamination Detection

Jeanne Moldenhauer

CONTENTS

6.1 INTRODUCTION

Environmental monitoring is an area of regulatory focus and has been for many years. There are several reasons for this, for example concerns that contamination present in the environment will have a high likelihood of contaminating the product being manufactured, concerns of increased risk of contamination in aseptic processes, loss of confidence in the ability of sterility tests to detect contamination, and so forth.

It has even been said that the environmental monitoring program is often used as a *de facto* sterility test. This is based upon the knowledge that the compendial sterility test was inherently flawed in its ability to determine product sterility (Moldenhauer and Sutton, 2004).

The situation is complicated by the fact that there are very few regulatory requirements for environmental monitoring. In most cases, the regulations cited for issues with environmental monitoring is 21CFR 211.113 "Control of microbiological contamination." This regulation states (FDA, 2017):

1. Appropriate written procedures, designed to prevent objectionable microorganisms in drug products not required to be sterile, shall be established and followed.
2. Appropriate written procedures, designed to prevent microbiological contamination of drug products purporting to be sterile, shall be established and followed. Such procedures shall include validation of all aseptic and sterilization processes.

Little guidance is provided in this regulation on how a program should be established. The most detailed regulatory expectations for environmental monitoring are provided in the FDA's Aseptic Processing Guidance (FDA, 2004). Since this is the most detailed description of a program, investigators have used its requirements as the expectation for all types of processes, including non-sterile products and terminally sterilized products. While some of the requirements are appropriate for all processes, in some cases this is definite overkill of what is needed. A common difference in the programs for different types of products is the number of samples taken for evaluation, the frequency of sampling, and the limits applicable to the process (Moldenhauer, 2017a).

Another problem that frequently occurs is that when limits are based upon room classifications, e.g., ISO 5, 7, or 8, investigators frequently look at the microbiological limits in the FDA's Aseptic Guidance. It is important to note that using the ISO classification system, there are no microbiological limits established in ISO 14644-1 (ISO, 2015). The ISO document bases cleanroom classifications solely on the nonviable particulate levels (Moldenhauer, 2017a).

Due to these types of issues, it becomes critical that the subject matter experts (SMEs) at your site clearly know the regulations and can accurately and clearly explain these differences in requirements.

6.2 A COMPLETE ENVIRONMENTAL MONITORING PROGRAM – WHAT DOES IT ENCOMPASS?

There are many different components of an environmental monitoring program. The Parenteral Drug Association's (PDA) Technical Report Number 13 (Revised) identified more than twenty different components of this type of program (PDA, 2014). These components go beyond the media, samples taken, getting results, and comparing the results to established limits. Some of the components of this type of program include (Moldenhauer, 2017a):

- A contamination control program that has identified the necessity of an environmental monitoring program and how it should be implemented.
- An environmental monitoring master plan.
- An environmental monitoring oversight committee (in some companies this is may be part of a sterility assurance committee or a contamination control committee).
- Selected laboratory methods and equipment:
  - Qualified equipment
  - Qualified methods
  - Selection of sample sites based upon risk assessment
  - Validation/qualification of the incubation and media conditions utilized.
- Microbiological methods specifically for collection of samples from: water, air, compressed gases, surfaces, personnel, and clean steam as appropriate.
- Appropriate method suitability testing results for all methods utilized.
- Conduct of installation qualification (IQ) and operational qualification (OQ) of the manufacturing equipment, and testing equipment utilized (e.g., RMMs) at least.
- Conduct of the environmental monitoring performance qualification (PQ). This data may be obtained.
- A risk assessment program to establish the environmental monitoring sites to monitor.
- Concurrent with media or water fills. As part of the final report, it is common to adjust or solidify the routine sampling sites to utilize based upon the data obtained in the PQ.
- Verification that all operators and technicians are trained and qualified for the tasks which they perform.
- Establishment of the routine environmental monitoring program.
- Specified monitoring methods and written procedures.
- Procedures for data collection, analysis, and trending. This step also includes the establishment of the appropriate limits or levels for the process.

- Trending may include use of automated systems, which are qualified. If manual procedures are used, they should be clearly documented, specify which trends are recorded, how often reports should be generated, and who is responsible for the reporting, review, and approval.
- Investigation of microbial data deviations (MDD) and resolution of issues
- Identification of contaminants using qualified methods.
- Maintenance of a library of isolates for your facility
- Process for conducting a product impact analysis. For non-sterile products this may include concerns with the FDA Bad Bug List, depending upon the route of administration, and the PDA's Technical Report No. 67 (2014) on the Exclusion of Objectionable Organisms.
- Determination of the objectionable organisms listing for your products and facility.
- A change control program that evaluates changes for the impact on the system and whether validation is needed.
- A corrective and preventative action program (CAPA) that addresses the cause of the excursion and how it was fixed. Including a check of the effectiveness of the program.

This type of program is depicted in Figure 6.1.

6.3   ARE THERE GAPS IN YOUR PROGRAM?

Established companies probably set up their monitoring program several years ago. One of the problems that frequently occurs is a failure to look at whether your program meets today's regulatory requirements. As such, we tend to shelve the program and only revise or update it when we have adverse regulatory investigations. These types of programs should be living documents that are reviewed and updated on a periodic basis to reflect current regulatory expectations.

6.4   THE ENVIRONMENTAL MONITORING COMMITTEE

The purpose of the environmental monitoring committee, whether it is an independent group or part of another committee is to ensure that senior management is aware of what is happening in the environmental monitoring program at the site. The intent of this management involvement is an expectation that an assessment will occur to determine whether the facility is operating within a state of control, whether policies or practices need to change, whether corrective actions have been effective, and the like. It can also be useful to obtain the necessary financial support to make lasting changes due to monitoring issues (Moldenhauer, 2017b).

This committee should be a cross-functional team, with high-level representatives from the various disciplines. At minimum, management level individuals from quality, operations, validations, quality control laboratories, and product development should be included. Other disciplines may be needed for specific meetings, e.g., medical representatives to aid in understanding risks associated with objectionable organisms (Moldenhauer, 2017b).

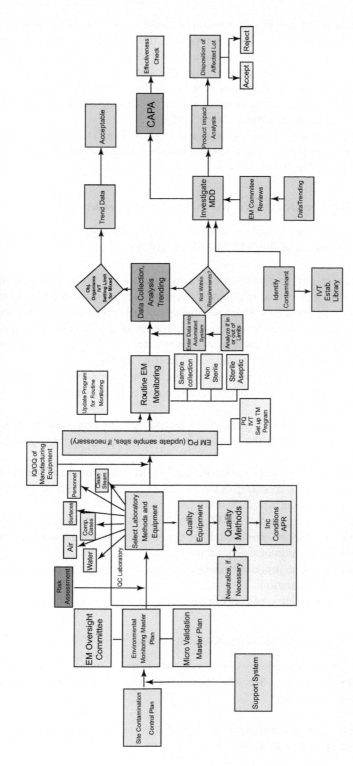

FIGURE 6.1 Environmental Monitoring Program.

It is critical that part of this committee's responsibility is the assurance that senior management is aware of what is happening in the plant regarding this program. It is also important that this committee ensure that appropriate product impact assessments are conducted when a contamination event occurs. The assessments should be reviewed to ensure that they are scientifically sound and appropriate. As regulatory expectations change, this committee should be driving the site's compliance to the changing requirements (Moldenhauer, 2017b).

Another function of this committee is to provide an assessment of the appropriateness and effectivity of the employee training programs relative to environmental monitoring (Moldenhauer, 2017b).

6.4.1 Types of Documents Reviewed by the Committee

The following is an example of some of the types of issues considered or documents reviewed by the committee (Moldenhauer, 2017b):

- Periodic environmental monitoring trending reports. (Most companies meet at least quarterly. Monthly meeting may be warranted for sterile processes or processes under regulatory scrutiny. The appropriate frequency is somewhat dependent upon the frequency of monitoring in the facility.)
- Changes in disinfectant effectiveness due to changes in environmental flora, new cleanroom surfaces, or cleaning agents.
- Quality metrics that provide information on the number of excursions, failures to meet alert and action levels, types of isolates recovered in the facility, and the like.
- Information on the types of corrective actions that have been taken to address the issues that have occurred in the program during the current evaluation period.
- Proposals for system changes that could affect environmental monitoring, e.g., work orders, re-modeling of the facility or specific work areas, and so forth.
- Changes in contracted cleaning companies.
- Changes in equipment used for monitoring and/or frequencies of use.
- Risk assessments conducted for the environmental monitoring program and/or validation of the system.
- Summaries of product impact assessments conducted during the period under consideration.
- Other information of concern regarding environmental monitoring.

6.4.2 Managing the Environmental Monitoring Committee

In most cases, the quality assurance department manages the environmental monitoring committee. Some of the responsibilities of quality assurance include (Moldenhauer, 2017b):

- Ensuring that the appropriate departments submit the documentation to be reviewed at the meeting.

- Setting up the meetings at the specified frequency.
- Moderate the meetings.
- Invite higher levels of senior management, when deemed appropriate. Alternatively, they are responsible for ensuring that senior management is made aware of issues.
- Ensure that trending reports are generated in accordance with approved procedures and reviewed in each meeting.
- Issuing meeting minutes to the committee members and affected personnel throughout the facility.

6.4.3 WHAT TYPE OF OUTPUTS SHOULD COME FROM THE ENVIRONMENTAL MONITORING COMMITTEE?

The committee should have several outputs. For example (Moldenhauer, 2017b):

- Meeting minutes for each meeting.
- Summaries of the data generated should be included in the senior management reports.
- Notification of issues to the affected departments of ongoing environmental trends.
- Immediate notification to senior management of new incidents of objectionable organisms, pathogenic organisms, and the like.

6.4.4 RESPONSIBILITY OF THE COMMITTEE

One of the key responsibilities of this committee is to ensure that "real" corrective actions are taken to resolve environmental monitoring issues. Also, the committee should ensure that the appropriate product impact assessments are conducted to ensure that product batches have been appropriately reviewed before release following a deviation. Part of this responsibility involves ensuring that the appropriate functional groups (at the right level) are involved in the decision-making (Moldenhauer, 2017b).

6.5 THE MICROBIOLOGICAL MASTER PLAN

Companies have been developing site master plans and/or validation master plans for many years. In more recent years, there has been a movement to either ensuring that these plans include significant information on microbiology or that a separate microbiology master plan has been established (Moldenhauer, 2017b).

The microbiology master plan (whether separate or part of another document) should provide the requirements for the following (Moldenhauer, 2017a):

- Details of how methods are selected and whether they need to be validated or qualified.
- Requirements for qualification of equipment and software in the laboratory.

- Descriptions of how equipment is selected, qualified, and implemented.
- Description of the change control program.
- Outlines the laboratory's entire operation.

6.6   RISK ASSESSMENTS TO DETERMINE
THE SAMPLING LOCATIONS

There is a regulatory expectation that risk assessment be conducted to determine the sampling sites to use for viable and non-viable monitoring in pharmaceutical facilities. While this expectation exists, there is no clear guidance on how this should be accomplished. There are a variety of different approaches available for use, and while this method is provided as guidance, it is not the only approvable method. It is important that you can explain why you chose the method you use and what is the basis for this method of selection.

6.6.1   How Many Sample Sites Should Be Selected?

Many have the misconception that if sampling locations are based upon risk, one can select a single sampling location in a room for routine monitoring. While this sounds reasonable based upon risk, it is unlikely that you will be successful in convincing a regulatory investigator that this is a sufficient number of sampling locations, especially for an aseptic process.

The number of sampling locations to utilize, during qualification should be determined based upon the test type and surface being sampled (Sutton, 2009).

Typical sample sites include:

- Non-viable air sampling (particulates)
- Active air sampling (airborne viables)
- Passive sampling of airborne viables (settle plates)
- Surface sampling (walls and floors)
- Surface sampling (equipment)

6.6.1.1   Non-Viable Particulates

ISO 14644-1 (2015) provides guidance on the selection of sampling locations for non-viable particulate monitoring, which is the defined scope of the document (Sutton, 2009). This following calculation is provided:

$$N_L = \sqrt{A}$$

Where N_L is the minimum number of sampling locations (rounded up to a whole number); and

A is the area of the clean room or zone in meters^2

6.6.1.2   Viable Active Air Sampling

Sutton (2009) makes a case for the conduct of both viable and non-viable active air sampling being conducted at the same location (or as close as practical to avoid compromising the other measure, or integrity of the product). If this approach is utilized, then both the number of sampling locations for viable active air sampling and non-viable particulates are the same.

6.6.1.3   Passive Air Sampling (Settle Plates)

Today, many regulatory documents expect that passive air sampling will be conducted. Some even believe that these samples are the best indicator of what is happening in the environment, as it mimics how contamination may "fall onto" the product. Another benefit of passive sampling is that the plates may be exposed for up to four hours continuously. The length of exposure should be qualified with growth promotion testing at the beginning and end of the exposure period.

The ideal placement of passive sampling plates is very near product exposure points. Sutton (2009) indicates that a similar number of settle plates be used as those used for active air sampling. The sampling locations are not likely to be the same.

6.6.1.4   Surface Samples

None of the regulatory guidance is geared to describe the number of sample sites for surface samples. One method that has been successfully used is to utilize the guidance in ISO 14644-1 (2015) for non-viable particulates for surface samples. In this case, each type of surface would be treated separately, and the minimum number of samples based upon the square root of its surface area. This works well for walls and floors (Sutton, 2009).

The number of equipment surface samples should be based upon the type of equipment utilized and the manufacturing process. There are no specific rules for how to determine this number. Your rationale should be documented so that you can easily explain the rationale to an investigator.

6.6.2   WHERE SHOULD I SAMPLE?

As with many topics in environmental monitoring, there is no specific guidance on where to sample. PDA Technical Report No. 13 (Revised) (2014) provides some useful guidance on selection of sample sites, for example:

Factors to consider in selecting sites for routine surveillance are:

- At which sites would microbial contamination most likely have an adverse effect on product quality?
- What sites would most likely demonstrate heaviest microbial proliferation during actual production?
- Should site selection involve a statistical design or should site selection be made on the basis of grid profiling? Should some sites for routine monitoring be rotated?
- What sites would represent the most inaccessible or difficult areas to clean, sanitize, or disinfect?
- What activities in the area contribute to the spread of contamination?
- Would the act of sampling at a given site disturb the environment sufficiently to cause erroneous data to be collected or contaminate product?

Additional guidance is provided in the FDA's Aseptic Processing Guidance document (FDA 2004) also provides some guidance in section IVA:

- "Air in the immediate proximity of exposed sterilized containers/closures and filling/closing operations would be of appropriate particle quality when it has a per-cubic-meter particle count of no more than 3520 in a size range of 0.5 μm and larger when counted at representative locations normally not more than 1 foot away from the work site, within the airflow, and during filling/closing operations. This level of air cleanliness is also known as Class 100 (ISO 5)."
- "We recommend that measurements to confirm air cleanliness in critical areas be taken at sites where there is most potential risk to the exposed sterilized product, containers, and closures. The particle counting probe should be placed in an orientation demonstrated to obtain a meaningful sample. Regular monitoring ... should be performed during each production shift. We recommend conducting nonviable particle monitoring with a remote counting system. These systems are capable of collecting more comprehensive data and are generally less invasive than portable particle counters."
- "Some operations can generate high levels of product (e.g., powder) particles that, by their nature, do not pose a risk of product contamination. It may not, in these cases, be feasible to measure air quality within the one-foot distance and still differentiate background levels of particles from air contaminants. In these instances, air can be sampled in a manner that, to the extent possible, characterizes the true level of extrinsic particle contamination to which the product is exposed. Initial qualification of the area under dynamic conditions without the actual filling function provides some baseline information on the non-product particle generation of the operation."

Further on in section XA of the FDA's Aseptic Guidance (FDA, 2004) it says:

- "Sample timing, frequency, and location should be carefully selected based upon their relationship to the operation performed..."
- "It is important that locations posing the most microbiological risk to the product be a key part of the program. It is especially important to monitor the microbiological quality of the critical area to determine whether or not aseptic conditions are maintained during filling and closing activities. Air and surface samples should be taken at the locations where significant activity or product exposure occurs during production. Critical surfaces that come in contact with the sterile product should remain sterile throughout an operation. When identifying critical sites to be sampled, consideration should be given to the points of contamination risk in a process, including factors such as difficulty of setup, length of processing time, and impact of interventions."

The European GMPs provide some guidance for sample site selection in the document "Manufacture of Sterile Medicinal Products" (EU 2008):

- "18. Where aseptic operations are performed monitoring should be frequent using methods such as settle plates, volumetric air and surface sampling (e.g. swabs and contact plates). Sampling methods used in operation should not interfere with zone protection."

There is also some guidance in USP Chapter < 1116> (USP, 2007):

- "Microbiological sampling sites are best selected when human activity during manufacturing operations are considered. Careful observation and mapping of a clean room during the qualification phase can provide information concerning the movement and positioning of personnel within these rooms. Such observation can also yield important information about the most frequently conducted manipulations and interventions."
- "Other areas of concern relative to introduction of contamination into clean rooms are at entry points where equipment and materials move from areas of lower classification to those of higher classification. Therefore, areas within and around doors and airlocks should be included in the monitoring scheme."

Determining the actual locations to sample in a room require an understanding of the manufacturing process, material flow, and personnel flow. Some of the considerations for sample site selection include (Sutton, 2009):

- Contamination vectors (handles, control panels, doors, and the like). Additionally, it is important to understand for example how doors are opened, like using the shoulder, the handle, your butt, or other methods.
- High traffic areas.
- Personnel flow.
- Material flow.
- Waste flow.
- Surfaces that are difficult to disinfect and or hard to reach effectively.
- HVAC (for this, we are looking mostly at the returns).
- Product risk.
- Extent of product exposure.
- The type of activity performed near that site.
- The potential for contaminations from interventions and manipulations.
- Contamination vectors.

The results of this selection process should be documented and appropriately approved.

Some companies prefer to utilize failure mode and effects analysis (FMEA) or hazard analysis critical control points (HACCP) to assess the risk associated with each potential sampling location. Other companies choose to write a technical justification explaining the risks and sampling locations selected based upon these risks. Any of these approaches can be acceptable.

6.7   DEVELOPING TEST METHODS

By definition, methods specified in the USP are considered validated. If these methods are utilized, they must be tested (qualified) to show method suitability at your site with your equipment, people, and supplies. If the methods are not compendial, the site is responsible for validation of the test method.

Many of the methods utilized for environmental monitoring are classical methods from the time of Pasteur and Koch. However, there are newer rapid or alternative microbiological methods. If these newer methods are used, there are several guidance documents available for how specifically to validate these methods, for example: USP < 1223>, EP 5.1.6 (EP, 2017) and the PDA's Technical Report No. 33 (Revised). The requirements for validation differ depending upon the type of test method, e.g., qualitative or quantitative. Separate requirements for identification systems are included in USP < 1113>.

6.8   SELECTING THE APPROPRIATE INCUBATION CONDITIONS AND MEDIA

There are regulatory expectations for companies to justify the media and incubation conditions utilized. An older version of USP < 1116 > provided for use of two different incubation conditions including 20°C–25°C and 30°C–35°C. When the USP < 1116 > chapter was updated to be applicable to aseptic processes only, the wording was changed to:

- "Time and incubation temperatures are set once the appropriate media have been selected. Typically, for general microbiological growth media such as SCDM, incubation temperatures in the ranges of approximately 20°C–35°C have been used with an incubation time of not less than 72 hours" [1]. With a 15°C range in temperature, it is not likely that a single study will provide adequate data to justify the incubation conditions use. As such, companies need to generate data to support the incubation conditions utilized."

6.8.1   HISTORICAL APPROACHES

Pharmaceutical companies have historically used two different media for conducting monitoring of the environment. One of the media was designed for the recovery of bacteria (typically trypticase soy agar or soybean casein digest agar) and the other was chosen to isolate fungi (mold and yeast). Frequently agars like potato dextrose agar or sabouraud dextrose agar are used for fungal recovery. The bacterial media was incubated at 30°–35°C for a specified number of days and the fungal media was incubated at 20°–25°C for a specified number of days (Moldenhauer, 2014).

Marshall et al. (1998) published an article entitled "Comparative Mold and Yeast Recovery Analysis (The Effect of Differing Incubation Temperature Ranges and Growth Media)." The paper described the studies performed to support the use of a single type of media to isolate both bacteria and fungi under a specified set of conditions that included two different temperature ranges (Moldenhauer, 2014).

As a part of evaluating a novel sterility test method, Kielpinski *et al.* (2005) studied the appropriate incubation temperature to use. Their data indicated that an incubation temperature of 32°C provided improved detection of the microorganisms in the sterility test method over the values obtained using the incubation conditions in the compendia (Moldenhauer, 2014).

USP < 1116> (USP, 2013) "Microbiological Control and Monitoring of Aseptic Processing Environments" indicates that when using two-temperature incubation of environmental monitoring plates, if one chooses to incubate at the lower temperature first, the recovery of Gram-positive cocci may be compromised. These are important as they are associated with humans, i.e., typical human contaminants.

As if the incubation temperature alone is not a big influence, there are also different types of media that may be used for recovery. The media used may contain neutralizing agents, like polysorbate 80 (Tween 80) and/or lecithin to improve the recovery of microorganisms from areas that may have been exposure to sanitizers or other antimicrobial substances (Moldenhauer, 2014).

Other concerns with environmental monitoring include: whether or not anaerobic monitoring should be conducted routinely, whether different culture media should be utilized, whether the incubation conditions selected can recover slow-growing microorganisms, and so forth (Moldenhauer, 2014).

6.8.2 A Protocol to Justify Incubation Conditions Used

A two-phase approach can be used to justify the environmental monitoring conditions. In this approach, Phase One involves testing a variety of samples in the laboratory to select an appropriate media and set of incubation conditions to evaluate in Phase Two. Phase Two is a comparative side-by-side study *in situ* looking at the existing environment monitoring conditions used, and the proposed monitoring method selected (Moldenhauer, 2014).

6.8.2.1 Phase One – Laboratory Testing

The purpose of Phase One testing is to establish the test conditions to evaluation in side-by-side testing. This testing allows for evaluation of various growth conditions, media, and recovery times. Consideration should be taken to determine the various types of organisms and media conditions to be evaluated. Test organisms should include both laboratory stock cultures and environmental isolates from the facility. A rationale should be prepared to identify how organisms were selected (there is no right or wrong way, but you should have a rationale and should include environmental isolates or stressed bugs), An example of a rational might be: use of at least one each of a Gram-positive cocci and bacillus, a Gram-negative cocci and bacillus, a mold and yeast. Additionally, prominent organisms previously isolated in environmental monitoring should be utilized. It is important to include a slow-growing microorganism (e.g., a microaerophilic) like *P. acnes* in the test scheme. You may choose to include more organisms of a specific type that are routinely found in the environment, or have been associated with adverse trends or sterility failures (Moldenhauer, 2014).

If you have an existing environmental monitoring program established, it may be beneficial to include those conditions routinely used in the test environment, especially if you intend to have acceptance criteria that compares to that same data (Moldenhauer, 2014).

This type of protocol can also be utilized to compare the differences in types of media. Additionally, you may wish to check the growth with and without neutralizers.

It is important to identify the various incubation conditions (temperature and time to be evaluated, e.g., 20°–25°C for three days followed by 30°–35°C for an additional three days or continue to incubate for up to seven, 30°–35°C for three days followed by 20°–25°C for an additional three days, 20°–25°C for up to seven days (final incubation time to be determined at the end of Phase One testing), 30°– 35°C for up to seven days (final incubation time to be determined at the end of Phase One testing), and so forth. For slow-growers, it is important that you consider time periods up to seven days to ensure that sufficient time has been provided for these organisms to grow (Moldenhauer, 2014).

Once the test parameters have been established, a series of studies are designed where each test organism is tested on each media for each of the indicated incubation conditions. For the extended incubation periods, such as up to seven days, it is worthwhile to record the counts daily to determine the optimal time for recovery of all specified organisms. While this is an extensive test, it provides a wealth of information for the facility (Moldenhauer, 2014).

The number of replicates to run for each test condition should also be specified. A higher number of replicates can be useful if using statistical analysis for the data (Moldenhauer, 2014).

One of the difficult aspects of the protocol is the determination of acceptance criteria, e.g., which set of conditions is best and why. In many cases, a company may want to use a single media and a single set of incubation conditions due to the cost benefits. This can be acceptable, providing that you do not overlook things like how long it took to recover slow-growing organisms (Moldenhauer, 2014).

It can be difficult to determine what level of recovery is required and what level is "equivalent." There is guidance in some different documents, but it is important to select a method and describe where it originated. You also need to identify whether all the test organisms need to be recovered, e.g., slow-growers, environmental isolates, anaerobes, and so forth.

6.8.2.2   Phase Two – Comparative study

Once the test conditions have been identified in Phase One, e.g., media, incubation time, and incubation temperature, the selected conditions will be tested *in situ*. If the company already has been using a different set of test conditions, the existing conditions may be tested concurrently to evaluate which method is better.

In these studies, the routine environmental monitoring is conducted using the optimum method selected in Phase One and the comparative method (old method). The samples are incubated and the data evaluated (Moldenhauer, 2014).

If a reference method is not available for comparison, the test method should be used *in situ* for a specified number of days much like one might do with an initial performance qualification of an environmental monitoring program (Moldenhauer, 2014).

6.9 SETTING ACTION AND ALERT LEVELS

For aseptic processes, most of the regulatory guidance documents have established acceptable action levels for many types of monitoring. Alert levels, however, are usually based upon historical values obtained. For example, if particulate monitoring requires an action level of 10,000 particles or less of the appropriate size, one might want to set an alert level at a number like 7,000 or 8,000 particles. The problem occurs if the actual data centers around 1,000 particles. It is better to select a limit based upon the actual values seen.

For non-sterile operations and terminal sterilization processes, it may be a bit more difficult to set action and alert levels. While it may be attractive to use statistical methods, one needs to ensure that the appropriate statistical methods are used. In most cases, the "cleaner" the area, the less likely it is for the data to be normally distributed.

Another issue is that for some non-sterile operations, monitoring may be conducted infrequently, e.g., monthly or quarterly. As such, it may be difficult to generate enough data to use a statistical method. It is important that the microbiologists work with any other groups aiding in the setting of levels.

6.10 DETERMINING THE OBJECTIONABLE ORGANISMS

For sterile processes (aseptic and terminally sterilized) the presence of any microorganisms in the product following sterilization is considered objectionable. It does not matter the type of organism, nor does the number of organisms present affect the determination of objectionable.

For non-sterile products there is a significant amount of guidance provided, e.g., USP < 1115> (USP, 2018), the Parenteral Drug Association's Technical Report No. 67 Exclusion of Objectionable Microorganisms from Non-sterile Pharmaceuticals, Medical Devices, and Cosmetics, (PDA, 2014) and other published literature.

6.11 QUALIFYING YOUR ENVIRONMENTAL MONITORING PROGRAM

There are different ways to qualify the environmental monitoring program. Some companies choose to qualify this program individually, while others may qualify this program along with the cleaning and disinfection process. Still other companies perform one comprehensive performance qualification for the entire aseptic process, including media fills, HVAC systems, and the like.

Key components of the qualification involve: taking samples *in situ*, before and after cleaning to evaluate whether the methods and procedures used will result in data that is within limits. Systems should be developed to ensure that the data is appropriately collected, entered and trended. There are several automated systems available to aid in this process. It is important that the data generated be reviewed in a variety of formats, e.g., where contamination is found in the facility, where specific isolates have been found in the facility, where results are within and outside of established limits, and so forth (Moldenhauer, 2017).

Ideally, this qualification should include both static and dynamic conditions. Sufficient replicates should be conducted to evaluate the effectiveness of the sites and the associated monitoring sites. For example, which sites are most likely to have contamination and how high is that contamination (Sutton, 2009).

6.12 SELECTING ROUTINE SAMPLING LOCATIONS

Ideally, sufficient data is available from the qualification runs to evaluate and determine the appropriate sampling locations for routine sampling. These sampling sites may be the same as the qualification, may be fewer sites, or may be totally different sampling plans. When selecting the routine sampling plan, it is important to note that it is NOT SUFFICIENT to select a single "worst-case" location for monitoring, especially in aseptic areas. The sampling locations should be documented along with a rationale for why they were selected. This justification should also include how many samples are required for each clean area or zone.

The FDA's Aseptic Processing Guidance (FDA, 2004) provides some guidance in section X.1.A, which states:

> All environmental monitoring locations should be described in SOPs with sufficient detail to allow for reproducible sampling of a given location surveyed. Written SOPs should also address elements such as (1) frequency of sampling, (2) when the samples are taken (i.e., during or at the conclusion of operations), (3) duration of sampling, (4) sample size (e.g., surface area, air volume), (5) specific sampling equipment and techniques, (6) alert and action levels, and (7) appropriate response to deviations from alert or action levels.

6.13 ESTABLISHING A LIBRARY OF ENVIRONMENTAL ISOLATES

There is an expectation of FDA to establish a list of the microorganisms commonly found in the aseptic facility. This is described in the FDA's Aseptic Guidance (FDA, 2004) section X.B.:

> Characterization of recovered microorganisms provides vital information for the environmental monitoring program. Environmental isolates often correlate with the contaminants found in a media fill or product sterility testing failure, and the overall environmental picture provides valuable information for an investigation. Monitoring critical and immediately surrounding clean areas as well as personnel should include routine identification of microorganisms to the species (or, where appropriate, genus) level. In some cases, environmental trending data have revealed migration of microorganisms into the aseptic processing room from either uncontrolled or lesser controlled areas. Establishing an adequate program for differentiating microorganisms in the lesser-controlled environments, such as Class 100,000 (ISO 8), can often be instrumental in detecting such trends. At minimum, the program should require species (or, where appropriate, genus) identification of microorganisms in these ancillary environments at frequent intervals to establish a valid, current database of contaminants present in the facility during processing (and to demonstrate that cleaning and sanitization procedures continue to be effective).

In recent years, this expectation has extended to other types of manufacturing processes. Additionally, many chapters of the USP as well as FD-483 observations and warning letters have stated a need to use environmental isolates when performing method suitability or qualification studies. There are several options for storing microorganisms, e.g., creation of "stock" cultures by microbiological isolate companies, creation of "bioball" cultures, low temperature freezing of cultures, and cryopreservation.

6.14   HANDLING MICROBIAL DATA DEVIATIONS

The "microbial data deviations" (MDD) procedure is a term coined by PDA to address microbial excursions from limits. This term was developed as most environmental data is not a specification, this term is better suited than the out-of-specification (OOS) used for most chemistry results. This type of procedure should require investigations into excursions, risk-based analysis of the results, analysis of the impact of the excursion on the product, and for non-sterile products should include concerns for whether there are specific concerns due to the type of contamination, i.e., objectionable organism. An organism that is always a concern is a member of the *Bacillus cereus* complex (BCC). This complex includes at least eighteen species of organisms are a concern by FDA for non-sterile aqueous preparations (Moldenhauer, 2017a).

An important function of this procedure is to determine the impact of the excursion on the product being manufactured. There is an expectation that quality assurance has the responsibility for assessing the appropriateness of product release.

6.15   CONDUCTING PRODUCT IMPACT ASSESSMENTS

The product impact analysis should be documented. Many consultants advise that it should be conducted via a written protocol. The document should discuss how decisions were made on the effect of this contaminant on the affected batch(es), and how the affected batch(es) were determined. Years ago, a common practice was to say something like, "the product passes sterility and endotoxin testing, so there is no product impact." These types of generic statements are not typically acceptable today. (Moldenhauer, 2017a) One of the big reasons for this is that the sterility test is not capable of assessing the risk of low level contamination in the batch. Many weaknesses of this test method have been described by Moldenhauer and Sutton (2004). Endotoxin testing is useful, but it is important to understand that for non-aqueous-based products the endotoxin may not be homogeneously distributed in the product tested. As such, contaminated product may not easily be found in "beginning, middle and end" samples.

The product impact assessment should be a written document that explains the various considerations made, explains the characteristics of the contaminating organisms and why it does or does not impact the product. There are some useful references that may aid in this process, e.g., FDA's Bad Bug Book available on the FDA website, or Medically Important Fungi (Moldenhauer, 2017a).

6.16   DOCUMENTATION

An extensive documentation system is required to support environmental monitoring, including: test procedures, sampling locations, media records, growth promotion records, testing results, calculations, environmental monitoring results, supporting automated system documentation, and the like.

6.17   ENVIRONMENTAL MONITORING IS A LIVING SYSTEM

It is important to recognize that this system is living, i.e., it should be routinely reviewed, and updated as appropriate. Sampling risks and contamination risks can change with the process. As such, periodic review and update is appropriate.

6.18   CONCLUSION

Environmental monitoring is a key component for ongoing assessment of the cleaning and disinfection processes being conducted at your facility. A well-designed program can provide useful information that may be used to aid in the upgrading and documentation of your system.

ACKNOWLEDGMENTS

This chapter is an expanded version of several articles published on the IVT Network. The articles are cited specifically in the Literature Cited section of this chapter.

LITERATURE CITED

EU (2008) EudraLex The Rules Governing Medicinal Products in the European Union. Volume 4: EU Guidelines to Good Manufacturing Practice Medicinal Products for Human and Veterinary Use: Annex 1 Manufacture of Sterile Medicinal Products.

EP (2017) 5.1.6 Alternative Methods for Control of Microbiological Quality. *European Pharmacopoeia* 9(2): 4339–4348. 07/2017:50111.

Food and Drugs Administration (2004) Guidance for Industry – Sterile Drug Products Produced by Aseptic Processing – Current Good Manufacturing Practice, Pharmaceutical cGMPs. United States Department of Health and Human Services, Center for Drug Evaluation and Research, Center for Biological Evaluation and Research, and the Office of Regulatory Affairs.

Food and Drugs Administration (2017) 21 CFR 211.113. Code of Federal Regulations Title 21. GMP Publications, Inc. www.gmppublications.com.

International Organization for Standardization (2015) ISO 14644–1:2015. Cleanrooms and Associated Controlled Environments.

Kielpinski, G., et al. (2005) Roadmap to Approval: Use of an Automated Sterility Test Method as a Lot Release Test for Carticel, Autologous Cultured Chondrocytes. *Cytotherapy* 7(6): 531–541.

Marshall, V., Poulson-Cook, S. and Moldenhauer, J. (1998) Comparative Mold and Yeast Recovery Analysis (The Effect of Differing Incubation Temperature Ranges and Growth Media). *PDA Journal of Pharmaceutical Science & Technology* 52(4): 166–169.

Moldenhauer, J. (2014) Justification of Incubation Conditions Used for Environmental Monitoring. *American Pharmaceutical Review Online*. Downloaded from: www.americanpharmaceuticalreview.com/Featured-Articles/158825-Justification-of-Incubation-Conditions-Used-for-Environmental-Monitoring/on January 24, 2017.

Moldenhauer, J. (2017a) Developing of Updating Your Environmental Monitoring Program to Meet Current Regulatory Expectations. Published on IVT Network. Downloaded from: www.ivtnetwork.com/article/developing-or-updating-your-environmental-monitoring-program-meet-current-regulatory-expecta on January 11, 2018.

Moldenhauer, J. (2017b) Establishing an Environmental Monitoring Oversight Committee. Downloaded from: www.ivtnetwork.com/article/establishing-environmental-monitoring-oversight-committee on January 17, 2018.

Moldenhauer, J. and Sutton, S. V. W (2004) Towards and Improved Sterility Test. *PDA Journal of Science and Technology* 58(6): 284–286.

Parenteral Drug Association (2014) Technical Report No. 13 (Revised) Fundamentals of an Environmental Monitoring Program. Bethesda, MD.

Parenteral Drug Association (2014) Technical Report No. 67 Exclusion of Objectionable Microorganisms from Nonsterile Pharmaceuticals, Medical Devices, and Cosmetics. Downloaded from: file:///C:/DocLib/PDA/Tech%20Reports/No%2067%20Exclusion%20of%20Objectionable%20Organisms.pdf on January 11, 2018.

Sutton, S. V. W. (2009) Qualification of an Environmental Monitoring Program – 1. Selection/Justification of Sample Sites. *PMF Letter*, August 2009. Downloaded from: www.microbiol.org/resources/monographswhite-papers/qualification-of-an-environmental-monitoring-program-1-selectionjustification-of-sample-sites/on January 24, 2018.

United States Pharmacopeia (2018) <1113> Microbial Characterization, Identification, and Strain Typing. Downloaded from: http://app.uspnf.com/uspnf/pub/index?usp=40&nf=35&s=2&officialOn=December 1, 2017 on January 29, 2018.

United States Pharmacopeia (2018) <1115> Bioburden Control of Nonsterile Drug Substances and Products. Downloaded from: http://app.uspnf.com/uspnf/pub/index?usp=40&nf=35&s=2&officialOn=December 1, 2017 on January 29, 2018.

United States Pharmacopeia (2013) <1116> General Chapters<1116>: Microbiological Control and Monitoring of Aseptic Processing Environments. Downloaded from http://www.uspnf.com/uspnf/pub/index?usp=36&nf=31&s=2&officialOn=December%201,%202013 on January 8, 2014.

United States Pharmacopeia (2018) <1223> Validation of Alternative Microbiological Methods. Downloaded from: http://app.uspnf.com/uspnf/pub/index?usp=40&nf=35&s=2&officialOn=December 1, 2017 on January 29, 2018.

7 Residue Removal in Cleanroom Environments

Jim Polarine and Beth Kroeger

CONTENTS

7.1 BACKGROUND

Although regulatory expectations and guidance documents indicate residue in cleanrooms is a concern for aseptic manufacturing and contamination control, often, those responsible for cleanroom environmental procedures fail to incorporate any type of routine rinsing or cleaning into their program. There still seems to be confusion and many opinions regarding cleaning, sanitization, disinfection, rotation, and rinsing. When rinsing is included in a program, it typically consists of rinsing for aesthetic reasons on materials where disinfectants leave a streaky residue, such as stainless steel, cleanroom curtains, glass, and mirrors. Floors and walls are neglected, and cleaning is frequently not performed. Accordingly, as these facilities age, deterioration and discoloration become more apparent from the lack of a robust program.

Not only can the presence of residue lead to issues with deterioration and discoloration, residues may impact the effectiveness of disinfectants used in the environment by essentially shielding the microorganism. Residues on stainless steel equipment may cause corrosion on equipment support structures, typically comprised of 304 stainless or 316 stainless steel. Clean, residue free surfaces are more easily monitored for these issues and then can be corrected before a larger issue arises.

Residues on cleanroom flooring can damage flooring substrates necessitating resurfacing or replacement. This is especially true with some of the newer flooring substrates that are common now. The surfaces of these substrates, while considered smooth, are quite rough. The flooring systems may range from having a slight texture to having aggregates incorporated into the flooring system intended to offer a degree of slip resistance to meet the needs of gowned operators wearing slick shoe covers. Consequently, residual detergents or process residues may build up in the depressions of the rough surface and discolor in a matter of weeks compared to smoother surfaces which may take up to a couple of months to show residual build-up. As such, equal concern should be given to residue removal as a preventive means to maintain the surfaces in the cleanroom.

Parenteral Drug Association (PDA) Technical Report 70, Fundamentals of Cleaning and Disinfection Programs for Aseptic Manufacturing Facilities, instructs to have a method for addressing residuals to ensure inspection readiness. "Due to their importance and direct impact on manufacturing operations, the cleaning and disinfection programs have been and continue to be a focus during regulatory inspections." [1]. This will continue to be an area for inspectional focus as cleaning and disinfection of rooms and equipment to produce aseptic conditions are frequently cited in warning letters and 21 CFR 211.42(c)(10)(v), relating to deficient cleaning systems, was ranked as the twelfth most issued inspectional observation in the last year reported [2].

The information provided in this chapter will clarify the regulatory expectations along with industry trends pertaining to residue removal in Cleanroom Environments. Additionally, application conditions leading to residues in the cleanroom are discussed and an *in situ* example of residue buildup and removal techniques are investigated using various cleaning agents and techniques for residue removal.

7.2   REGULATORY EXPECTATIONS AND GUIDANCE

The current industry regulations and guidance documents have several references related to residue control and rinsing strategies in cleanroom operations. The Pharmaceutical Inspection Convention (PIC) states the following regarding residues, "The cleaning procedure should also effectively remove product residues from surfaces of the workstation" [3]. ANVISA states the following "In the case of dedicated equipment, cleaning procedures used should be validated, considering residues of cleaning agents, microbiological contamination, and degradation products when applicable [4]. United States Pharmacopeia (USP) 40 General Chapter <1072> indicates the following: "Disinfectants applied on potential product contact surfaces are typically removed with 70% alcohol wipes. The removal of residual disinfectants should be monitored for effectiveness as a precaution against the possibility of product contamination"[5]. PDA Technical Report number 70 states the following: "The effect of buildup of residues, particles, and possibly microbes is also affected by the surface itself. Irregular or porous surfaces trap residues and other contaminants and make the surface more difficult to clean and disinfect. Development of an appropriate cleaning system is critical to successfully preparing a surface for disinfection. Cleaning operations should be performed routinely with frequency based on area, classification, usage, risk, and visible cleanliness" [6]. The current draft of Annex I indicates the following in relation to residue removal, "Cleaning programs should be effective in the removal of disinfectant residues" [7]. These recent regulatory guidance documents all emphasize residue is a significant concern in cleanrooms and on equipment surfaces. Therefore, having a program in place to control and mitigate residue build up in cleanroom environments can be considered an industry best practice.

Residues left on surfaces after cleaning and disinfection have been cited by Food and Drugs Administration (FDA) regulators. A recent FDA warning letter (483) stated the following, "Your response stated that the white residue on the face panel of the HEPA filter supplying air to the ISO 5 area was from disinfectant. However, you provided no documentation to support this statement and we remain concerned as it is not clear if you have removed the residue or evaluated the impact of this residue on product quality" [8].

Regulators are also concerned about the impact of residues on product quality. Recent FDA 483s have focused on residue left on cleanroom surfaces, "Specifically, during the inspection of your firm's cleaned equipment storage room, I observed a cleaned stainless-steel tray that had a visible, apparently sticky, crystallized white residue. Additionally, your firm's written procedure does not require visual inspection after major cleaning of the stainless-steel trays" [9]. Residues and residue build up needs to be controlled and addressed routinely to avoid citations from industry regulators.

7.3 WHY RESIDUE IS A MAJOR CONCERN

Residues from disinfectants, sanitizers, and sporicides must be periodically removed with either water-for-injection (WFI), 70% isopropyl alcohol (IPA), or a sterile cleaner. Residue build up over time can be a safety issue, functional issue, particle issue, efficacy issue, and an aesthetic issue. Residue may cause floors to be sticky, tacky, or slippery and can pose a risk to operator's safety. There have been instances where operators have had falls on cleanroom floors due to not rinsing residues from cleanroom surfaces. At a facility in Europe, residue from phenolics and sodium hypochlorite had not been removed in 12 years leaving the floors sticky which caused the operators shoes to stick to the floor. Residues can also pose a particulate risk in the cleanroom causing either an increase in particle levels or in some cases, getting onto cleanroom curtains and getting into drug products. Residues can build up and potentially hide microbes or even be a potential source of food for microbes leading to microbial proliferation in cleanrooms. The humidity and moisture in cleanrooms can even make residue a bigger issue in rare cases.

An issue our equipment cleaning counterparts are acutely aware of is corrosion on stainless steel surfaces caused by loss of the passive surface. "Passivation is the process by which a stainless steel surface will spontaneously form a chemically resistant surface when exposed to air or other oxygen-containing environments... providing that the surface has been thoroughly cleaned or descaled" [10]. Passivation will only occur on a surface that is thoroughly cleaned and free from residue, allowing the surface of the stainless steel contact with oxygen in air to form a protective chromium oxide enriched passive surface. When stainless steel loses its passive surface, either by surfactants remaining on the surface from cleaning agents or from surfaces routinely exposed to caustic disinfectants or oxidizing agents, corrosion may occur.

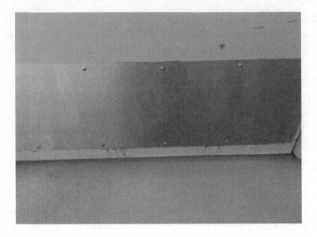

FIGURE 7.1   Corrosion on a stainless steel kick plate in a Class D area. Source: Kroeger, B. (2018) STERIS Corporation.

Figure 7.1 shows an example of rouge on a cleanroom surface resulting from frequent use of caustic disinfectants and oxidative chemistries without a proper residue removal procedure.

Severe corrosion may cause pitting on the surface of the stainless steel which may harbor microorganisms, shielded not only by the residue, but the corrosion, the surface, and potentially extracellular polymeric substances (EPS) found in biofilms. "The development and presence of the EPS is very important in increasing the micro-organisms resistance to environmental stresses, antimicrobial agents and cleaning agents" [11]. Any stainless steel in the environment should be rinsed after every application of antimicrobial or cleaning agent, not only for aesthetic reasons but to mitigate the formation of corrosion. This is especially true for ancillary cleanroom equipment such as the outside of laminar flow hoods, pumps, outside of autoclaves, sinks, racks, tables, chairs, mirrors, tank exteriors, benches, push plates, and garment stations.

7.4   DRAINS IN CLEANROOMS AND CONTROLLED AREAS

Drains are a consistent area of concern in cleanroom operations. Drains are locations where bioburden can grow and accumulate over time. *Pseudomonas*, *Burkholderia*, and other Gram-negative bacteria are common in drains and there have also been cleanroom operations where media has backed up into the drains and come out in the cleanroom. Corrosion is also a common issue with many drains. The PDA Technical Report 70 indicates the following, "Drains will most probably incorporate a biofilm on the inside of the drain that would prevent penetration of the disinfecting agent through the biofilm and from contacting the drain surface. Disinfecting the exterior of the drain's visible surface with sodium hypochlorite or peracetic acid and hydrogen peroxide may reduce bioburden, but such bioburden is expected to return within a short time period" [1]. FDA regulators have also highlighted drain areas as a potential area of concern as described in the FDA warning letter, "FDA collected environmental swabs during previous establishment inspection, revealing *L. monocytogenes* in three locations within your facility. Those locations included a dustpan handler, a floor drain and pooled water in corner" [12]. *Listeria monocytogenes*, which is a pathogen, has been a significant issue in the food and beverage industry as well [13].

The following are practical recommendations regarding drains in cleanrooms [14]:

- should be limited to Grade C and D areas
- are prohibited in Grade A/B areas (ISO 5)
- should be of adequate size
- must have air breaks between equipment/sinks and drains
- must have traps or water seals to prevent backflow
- must be capped, if possible (prevent effluent backup)
- must be shallow to facilitate cleaning and disinfection
- must be sampled and monitored around them
- must be cleaned and disinfected periodically

The cleaning frequency of drains varies from facility to facility, but the overall objective would be to keep bioburden low. Typically, drains should be cleaned weekly or monthly, but the frequency should be based on an assessment taking into consideration classification of area, use, and risk to process. Sodium hypochlorite, hydrogen peroxide, and hydrogen peroxide/peracetic acid blends are commonly used to control bioburden in drain areas. The best scenario would be to take the drain apart and soak the parts in a sporicide or disinfectant. Cleaning the drains with a neutral or acidic cleaner prior to using a sporicide would be optimal to remove any residues and build up around the drain prior to the disinfection step.

There may be situations where a formulated cleaner may be required to remove visual reside build up or hard to clean soils. If the drain is heavily soiled due to discarded process soils, biofilms, or rouge, a two or three-step approach may be necessary for remediation. A triple clean in this instance would consist of a pre-clean using a formulated neutral or alkaline detergent to remove any process residues and biofilm EPS followed by a formulated acidic detergent to remove any rouge followed with an application of a sporicidal agent or disinfectant using a product to target the microbes [15].

When handling drains, double gloving is recommended, so outer pair can be discarded after cleaning to avoid spreading contamination to other cleanroom surfaces. Care should be taken to avoid spreading residue and potential contamination by first sanitizing or disinfecting the top of any drain cover or cap. Remove any drain cover or standing drain pipe cap and sanitize or disinfect the underside as well as drain bowl or area around the drain. Parts removed from drain should be placed in a clean container or liner and not directly onto the cleanroom floor. For heavy residue, use of a formulated alkaline detergent may be necessary as well as elevated temperatures or mechanical action using a nylon brush. Any brush used should be at least one-half inch smaller than the diameter of the drain. Prepare approximately five liters of use-dilution. Decant at least one to two liters of cleaning solution down the drain.

Immerse brush into the cleaning solution and scrub using a circular or side-to-side motion until visually clean. When removing the brush from the drain, use care not to spatter to avoid contaminating adjacent surfaces. Place brush into a container or liner for contaminated items. Rinse the drain by sending water to the drain at a low pressure to prevent splashing. Follow cleaning by decanting at least one liter of a disinfectant or sporicidal agent into the drain including all sides of the drain bowl. Sanitize outer gloves and replace drain cover or cap. Place all material used to clean the drains and outer layer of gloves into the container or liner for contaminated items.

7.5   RESIDUE SOURCES

Residues in a cleanroom environment or aseptic processing area can originate from any number of sources since these spaces are used to manufacture product and not just meant to sit idle. The most understandable contributing cause of residues in the cleanroom result from daily application of disinfectants necessary to control the environment from microbial contamination. Any existing cleanroom lacking a rinsing or cleaning program will eventually have an issue with residues on the surfaces. These areas may have black residue on the floors and walls, white residue on any glass or dark color epoxy paint, and grey to white streaks on vinyl curtains and stainless steel. Eventually, stainless steel may begin to corrode as in the example of the kick plate in Figure 7.1. Dark colors in a cleanroom may be more susceptible to visible residue over light colors, much like a dark color car will show residue and spotting more than a light color vehicle. A recent trend in cleanroom design is to designate the area leading to or adjacent to fire safety equipment with red epoxy paint. This seems like it would be a worthwhile idea as it draws attention to the location of this equipment, but eventually, the continual use of oxidizing sporicidal agents will lead to white, hard to remove, streaks on the painted surface. For these areas, it is best to try to avoid dark colors, especially red. If the area is mandated to have this indication for safety requirements or the color is one where the color is inherited, a rinse may be required after every application of any oxidizing sporicidal agent after the required contact time. The same would be true for cleanrooms having many windows, stainless surfaces, and modular type cleanroom walls with extremely slick and reflective surfaces. Figure 7.2 demonstrates an external surface of a good manufacturing practice (GMP) washer where the residue was removed on the left side using isopropyl alcohol and residue from disinfectant application on the right side remaining on the surface.

Compatibility issues arising from the use of various agents in a rotation program may cause residues on surfaces. Standard industry practice for rotation consists of using one or more disinfectants along with a sporicide. Each disinfectant and cleaning agent is formulated with a specific and unique combination of ingredients designed to work together. Mixing the agents together, either in development of the "ultimate in-house cleaner" or from residual disinfectant from past applications mixing with a new application of a different product can potentially release harmful vapors or create an undesired reaction. Alternating between phenolic disinfectants and quaternary ammonium disinfectants without a thorough rinse in between is not recommended and highly discouraged. Cationic quaternary disinfectants may

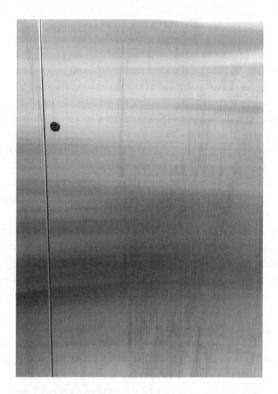

FIGURE 7.2 External surface of stainless steel equipment in a cleanroom. Source: Kroeger, B. (2018) STERIS Corporation.

contain non-ionic detergents which may inactivate phenolics. Anionic detergents present in anionic phenolic disinfectants may inactivate quaternary ammonium disinfectants. The actives in these two types of disinfectants may react with one another and form an insoluble residue. This typically will appear as a black, sticky residue on the surface.

Residues may also occur from poor cleaning practices such as overly concentrated use-dilutions prepared from concentrated cleaning agents. Sometimes more is not necessarily better. In one instance, a site was using a concentrated product at a dilution of seven parts formulated cleaner plus two parts organic solvent plus one-part WFI. Not only were they mixing different cleaning agents, the formulated product was intended to be used at a 1% concentration. The cleaning solution was sprayed directly onto the surface with no mechanical wiping and no rinsing after application. The materials of construction were glass, polycarbonate, and stainless steel. The residue formed on the surface was unable to be removed by any corrective measures since the surfaces were irrevocably damaged, ultimately requiring replacement.

Use of spent disinfectant solutions may also contribute to residues in the cleanroom. A spent solution is one where there are visible contaminants in the solution or the solution is used in an area after the recommended and validated liter/m^2 coverage area. Use-dilutions should have a defined and validated expiry and be discarded if there are visible contaminants in the disinfectant solution or after application to a defined surface area. Process soils may be spread from one area to another by contamination of the use-dilution. Typically, use-dilutions are changed out after every 93 m^2 in a Grade C or D area or when visibly dirty. A large corridor, such as a Grade D corridor in a facility, should be divided into grids and mopped with a corresponding bucket assembly prepared using fresh use-dilutions for every section of the grid to cover the entire surface area. These areas should be cleaned in a grid pattern and contact time measured for each area. Surface area in this instance is not how much solution in the bucket will cover the area, but rather, best practice on changing out a use-dilution to avoid using spent disinfectant solution. This should minimize spreading of process residues as they could interact with the disinfectant and/or contaminate the disinfectant. For heavy process residues, a pre-clean may be required using a cleaning agent such as WFI, ethanol/isopropyl alcohol, or a formulated detergent.

Since aseptic processing areas are manufacturing areas, as stated previously, drug product and process spills causing residue issues are more common than we like to admit. Even in the strictest bioprocessing environments, one may contend with ruptured hoses, buffer solutions containing salts and sugars draining out after a chromatography skid disconnection, leaking single-use bags, removal of unbled filters, and any number of incidents caused by the combination of high pressure systems and automation.

Large process spills may have to be pre-cleaned according to non-routine cleaning procedures and handled as a worse case event. When the environment is disrupted for any reason, processing operations should be suspended when safe to do so. Any in-process material should be reviewed by quality and a formal risk assessment or investigation performed to determine impact to the process/product and final disposition. The area should then be isolated by designating as out-of-service and the appropriate personnel notified. Personnel working in the area should be limited and if access is required, shoe covers should be used when entering or exiting the area to avoid contaminating the adjacent area. Clean the area impacted by the event by first clearing any spill or debris using a HEPA wet/dry vacuum or other appropriate means such as wipes, mops, or squeegees. After thoroughly cleaning the spill, triple clean the area with two applications of a disinfectant followed by a sporicidal agent [16].

There may be instances where the process spill itself or the combination of the drug product interacts with either disinfectant or process solutions resulting in difficult to remove residue or staining.

7.6   CASE STUDY: REMOVAL OF RESIDUE FROM DRUG PRODUCT INTERACTION WITH DISINFECTANT SOLUTION

A drug manufacturer encountered staining on the cleanroom floor in the production support area. The issue was believed to stem from the interaction of process residues and disinfectant solution. A study was performed testing concentrations of drug product and disinfectant solutions to determine the cause of stains and steps for remediation and prevention. Additionally, flooring substrates were tested to determine if one type of flooring was more resistant to staining. Flooring types tested were Sherwin-Williams #3744 CR Epoxy flooring, BASF #R61-SL Full Flake Epoxy, Sherwin-Williams #4685 100% Solid Urethane, and Sherwin-Williams PAce-Cote 4844.

The drug product was applied to each flooring sample under various disinfectant conditions to test potential root cause for staining. In the first condition, the drug product was applied to the surface of the flooring samples, dried under ambient conditions, and followed by an application of a phenolic disinfectant at the recommended use-dilution and then air dried under ambient conditions. For the second condition, the drug product was mixed with phenolic disinfectant at the recommended use-dilution, applied to the surface of the flooring coupons and then air dried under ambient conditions. Concentrated phenolic disinfectant was mixed with the drug product and applied to the surface of the flooring samples and air dried under ambient conditions as a third test condition. Lastly, the drug product was applied to the surface of each flooring sample and air dried under ambient conditions. Figure 7.3 depicts drug residue application under conditions described previously.

Several cleaning solutions were tested including a formulated alkaline detergent, a formulated alkaline detergent plus detergent additive, a detergent additive alone, a high-performance oxidative detergent, and an acidic detergent additive on each of the flooring coupons spiked with drug product and disinfectant after a seven-day dirty hold time at ambient temperature. Each section with four spots was then scrubbed with a nylon-bristled brush for not more than five minutes using one of the cleaning solutions described above at ambient temperature (20°C–25°C). Results indicate staining occurred when concentrated disinfectant was mixed with drug product. This seemed to coincide with observations at the site where it was noticed the heaviest staining occurred in the equipment cleaning area where use-dilutions of the disinfectant solution was prepared. Incidental spills of drug product and concentrated disinfectant were inadvertently mixing in this cleaning area causing the staining.

Use of alkaline solutions on the flooring substrates removed visible residues and staining but left the surfaces tacky. Use of a detergent additive alone and use of an oxidative detergent did not leave the surface of the flooring substrates tacky, however, an oxidative detergent was required to remove the residue from the surface of the flooring coupons using a 1% solution, ambient conditions with a one-minute dwell/scrub time followed by a rinse. Although the oxidative detergent could remove residue from the surface of all coupons, two of the flooring coupons, Sherwin-Williams #4685 100% Solid Urethane and Sherwin-Williams PAce-Cote 4844, had faint yellowish stains which remained. Both the visible residue and residual staining were able to be removed from Sherwin-Williams #3744 CR Epoxy flooring and BASF

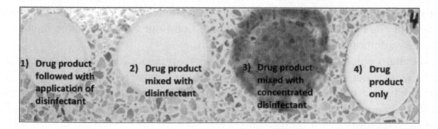

FIGURE 7.3 Flooring coupon spiked with drug product and various conditions of disinfectant to investigate staining root cause and corrective/preventive measures. Source: Johnston, C. and Lopolito, P. (2007) Process and Cleaning Evaluation (PACE®Evaluation).

#R61-SL Full Flake Epoxy flooring using 1% solution of oxidative detergent. It is important to note, the use of an acid after a formulated alkaline detergent did remove the tackiness of the flooring surface and did result in stain removal on the two flooring samples with faint yellow stains after cleaning with the oxidative detergent.

The take home message from the study is that drug product may cause residue issues and, in some cases, should be considered in a site's residue removal plan. Specifically, interaction may occur between drug product and sanitizing, disinfecting, or sporicidal agents, becoming harder to clean, particularly with concentrated product. If potential for process spills exist, a site may want to evaluate flooring types and cleaning capability of rinse agents to prevent staining and have a cleaning process established for these types of residues. Testing residue removal products (formulated cleaners) and effectiveness can be conducted outside of the cleanroom in a laboratory and may be valuable means to save resources.

7.7   RECOMMENDED PROCEDURE FOR RESIDUE REMOVAL

PDA Technical Report 70, Fundamentals of Cleaning and Disinfection Programs for Aseptic Manufacturing Facilities, section 9.0 describes cleaning as a "nondestructive mechanical action that loosens and removes contaminants from the area or equipment surface. Procedurally, a cleaning agent is applied via a nondestructive mechanical action method. Contaminants and residues are loosened and rinsed from the surface and removed with a squeegee or dry cloth." Section 2.0 describes types of cleaning agents by defining as "a solution or solvent used in the washing step of a cleaning process and lists examples as water, organic solvent, commodity chemical diluted in water and formulated detergent diluted in water." An ideal cleaning agent is formulated with an "effective surfactant system that will support the water in its efforts to release particles, residues and other foreign materials" [17].

7.8   RESIDUE REMEDIATION – AN *IN SITU* CASE STUDY

A sterile liquids manufacturer was considering floor resurfacing/replacement due to the state of their cleanroom surfaces. The two-year-old floors had visible residue resulting from daily application of a phenolic disinfectant and a once per month application of a sporicidal agent, without routine rinsing. The resulting black residue is shown in Figure 7.4. The site flooring system was a DESCO Quartz Epoxy flooring system, where the structure of the flooring system is designed to be not smooth to prevent slips. Thus, more solution remained on floor causing residue issues and ultimately, deterioration of the flooring system.

The main objective of the study was to compare a sterile oxidative detergent, a sterile neutral detergent, and sterile WFI ability to remove residual disinfectant and sporicidal agent build up from a floor in an ISO 8 aseptic area. The other objective was to determine the most appropriate manner to apply the cleaner for effectiveness in residue removal.

The DESCO flooring system was marked off in a grid pattern for *in situ* testing of various solutions' ability to remove the built-up residual combination of disinfectant and sporicidal agent from the floor. Images were taken to document the state of the

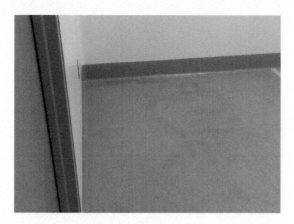

FIGURE 7.4 DESCO Quartz Epoxy flooring system, two years post install. Floors disinfected daily with phenolics and once per month application of sporicidal agent. Source: Kroeger, B. (2017) STERIS Corporation.

flooring prior to any residue removal attempts, Figure 7.5. Environmental sampling using RODAC® plates were taken in each grid in three separate locations before and after test to determine if removal of residue impacts environmental data. In addition, control samples were taken from random locations on the floor surface as routine monitoring samples before and after residue removal step.

The mop system, depicted in Figure 7.6, used for residue removal test was a Micronova™ Slim T™ double-bucket cart and Micronova™ Slimline™ wringer using a Micronova™ mop handle with a Micronova™ Slimline™ 14" mop adapter and Micronova™ Snap Mop PolySorb 14-inch irradiated covers, Figure 7.6.

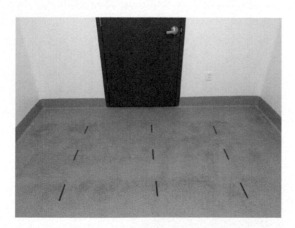

FIGURE 7.5 DESCO Quartz Epoxy flooring system in an ISO 8 cleanroom environment marked off in a grid pattern for *in situ* testing. Two-year-old floors are disinfected daily with phenolics and once per month application of sporicidal agent. Source: Kroeger, B. (2017) STERIS Corporation.

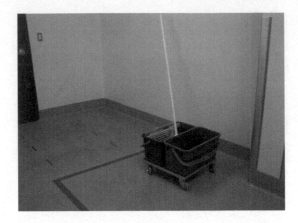

FIGURE 7.6 Micronova™ Slim T™ double-bucket cart and Micronova™ Slimline™ wringer assembly. Source: Kroeger, B. (2017) STERIS Corporation.

The floors were mopped in a back and forth pattern ten times to loosen the soil and the results were captured in images prior to any removal of the detergents using sterile WFI. Figure 7.7 shows the DESCO flooring after residue removal using WFI to clean lane one, a sterile oxidative detergent in lane two, and a sterile neutral detergent in lane three. Figure 7.8 is an image of lane one prior to residue removal and Figure 7.9 is the same lane after use of WFI to remove residue. Figure 7.10 is an image of lane two prior to residue removal and Figure 7.11 is the same lane after use of a sterile oxidative detergent to remove residue. Figure 7.12 is an image of lane three prior to residue removal and Figure 7.13 is the same lane after use of a sterile neutral detergent.

The *in situ* results for residue removal indicate the sterile neutral detergent used in lane three was the better option for removing residual disinfectant and sporicidal

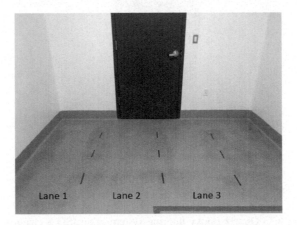

FIGURE 7.7 DESCO flooring after residue removal trial using WFI (lane 1), a sterile oxidative detergent (lane 2), and a sterile neutral detergent (lane 3). Source: Kroeger, B. (2017) STERIS Corporation.

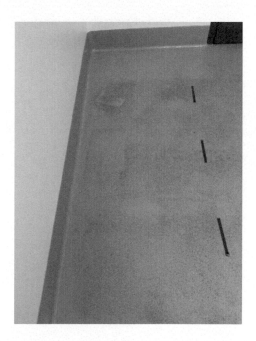

FIGURE 7.8 DESCO flooring before (image on left) and after residue removal (image on right) using WFI. Source: Kroeger, B., (2017) DESCO flooring prior to residue removal test with WFI.

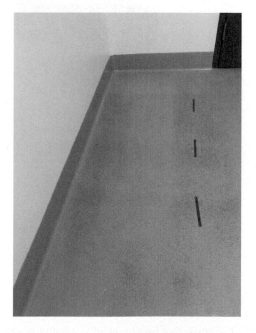

FIGURE 7.9 DESCO flooring before (image on left) and after residue removal (image on right) using WFI. Source: Kroeger, B., (2017) DESCO flooring after residue removal test with WFI.

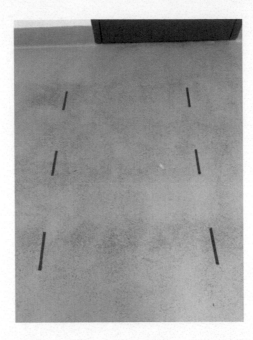

FIGURE 7.10   DESCO flooring before (image on left) and after residue removal (image on right) using sterile oxidative detergent. Source: Kroeger, B., (2017) DESCO flooring prior to residue removal test using sterile oxidative detergent.

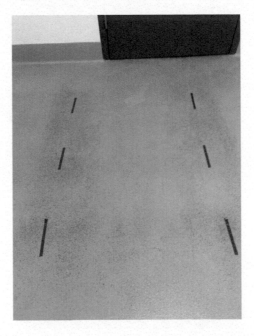

FIGURE 7.11   DESCO flooring before (image on left) and after residue removal (image on right) using sterile oxidative detergent. Source: Kroeger, B., (2017) DESCO flooring after residue removal test using sterile oxidative detergent.

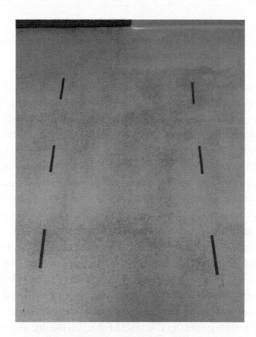

FIGURE 7.12 DESCO flooring before (image on left) and after residue removal (image on right) using sterile neutral detergent. Source: Kroeger, B., (2017) DESCO flooring prior to residue removal test using sterile neutral detergent.

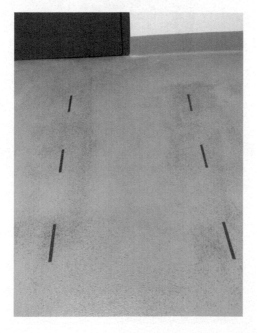

FIGURE 7.13 DESCO flooring before (image on left) and after residue removal (image on right) using sterile neutral detergent. Source: Kroeger, B., (2017) DESCO flooring after residue removal test using sterile neutral detergent.

agents, under the conditions tested, those being mopping in a back and forth pattern ten times using 1% use-dilution. Comparable results were obtained using sterile oxidative detergent, however, the oxidative solution required a five-minute contact time. Once a thorough cleaning has been completed, a routine rinsing program using alcohol or WFI should be sufficient to maintain low residue levels. As with the disinfectants, where the environment is routinely monitored to demonstrate bioburden control, cleanroom surfaces should be monitored to ensure residue levels are under control. We recommend rinsing quarterly to biannually and increasing frequency based on residue levels and/or environmental control. Typically, cleanrooms are rinsed at least monthly with surfaces more at risk for residual impact, such as stainless steel, rinsed after application of disinfectant or sporicidal agent.

The cleaner should be applied in a manner that is not in alignment with typical application of a disinfectant, i.e. using unidirectional, overlapping strokes. The objective of the cleaning step is to loosen soil on the surface so mechanical action is preferred using circular motion with approved cleaning utensils that are compatible with the cleaner, Figure 7.14. Cleaned surfaces are then rinsed using WFI or purified water. Figure 7.15 shows the DESCO Quartz Epoxy flooring system after residue removal using sterile neutral detergent and subsequent rinse to remove detergent. As can be seen from the image, the floors are nearly restored to their post-install condition thus negating the need for resurfacing at a fraction of the cost and lost time.

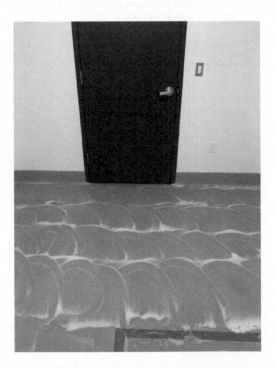

FIGURE 7.14 Application of sterile neutral detergent. Source: Kroeger, B. (2017) STERIS Corporation.

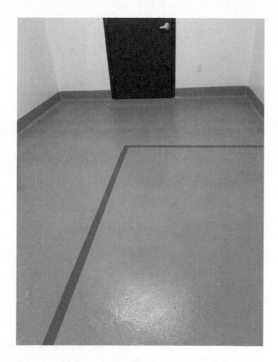

FIGURE 7.15 DESCO flooring after residue removal trial using sterile neutral detergent and rinse. Source: Kroeger, B. (2017) STERIS Corporation.

Close-up images were taken both before and after residue removal to emphasize the residue deposited in the depressions of the textured flooring system. Figure 7.16 shows a close-up image of the residue on the floor prior to cleaning and Figure 7.17 shows a close-up image of the floor after cleaning using a 1% solution of a sterile neutral detergent. These images demonstrate the detergent's ability to loosen the residue and lift it from the surface of the cleanroom floor to restore the surface to its expected state.

The results of the environmental sampling using RODAC® plates were interesting. Samples were taken in each grid or lane in three separate locations before and after cleaning, prior to any disinfection. Table 7.1 represents the environmental monitoring results prior to and post residue removal using WFI; Table 7.2 represents the environmental monitoring results prior to and post residue removal using sterile oxidative detergent; Table 7.3 represents the environmental monitoring results prior to and post residue removal using sterile neutral detergent; and Table 7.4 represents the environmental monitoring control sample results prior to and post residue removal.

Overall, there were slightly less organisms after cleaning in the lanes where detergents were used compared to the use of WFI. The number of organisms detected in the WFI grid floor surface increased slightly after cleaning. Prior to cleaning, the most prevalent organisms were species of bacillus (*B.subtilis, B. arybhattai, B. amyloliquefaciens,* and *B.licheniformis*), staphylococcus (*S. sarprohyticus* and *S. cohnii*), and micrococcus. After cleaning, there were predominantly staphylococcus (*S. epidermidis*) and bacillus species.

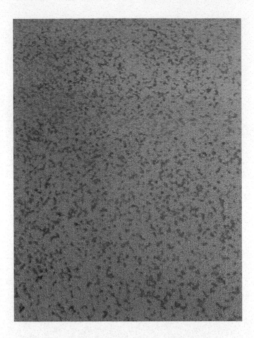

FIGURE 7.16 Close-up image of DESCO flooring after two years of residue buildup (image on left) and close-up image of DESCO flooring after cleaning with sterile neutral detergent (image on right). Source: Kroeger, B. (2017) STERIS Corporation.

FIGURE 7.17 Close-up image of DESCO flooring after two years of residue buildup (image on left) and close-up image of DESCO flooring after cleaning with sterile neutral detergent (image on right). Source: Kroeger, B. (2017) STERIS Corporation.

TABLE 7.1

Environmental monitoring sample results, prior to and post residue removal using WFI

WFI Results					
Before Cleaning			After Cleaning		
EM Sample ID	Results cfu/plate	Microbial Isolates	EM Sample ID	Results cfu/plate	Microbial Isolates
1A1	<1	N/A	1A2	5	*M. luteus* *S. epidermidis*
2A1	3	*B. subtilis* *S. sarprohyticus*	2A2	6	*S. epidermidis*
3A1	5	*B. subtilis*	3A2	5	*Paenibacillus lentus*

Source: Kroeger, B. (2017) STERIS Corporation.

TABLE 7.2

Environmental monitoring sample results, prior to and post residue removal using Sterile oxidative detergent

Sterile oxidative detergent					
Before Cleaning			After Cleaning		
EM Sample ID	Results cfu/plate	Microbial Isolates	EM Sample ID	Results cfu/plate	Microbial Isolates
1B1	10	*B. arybhattai*	1B2	3	*O. kimchi*
2B1	13	*M. luteus*	2B2	4	*B. amyloliquefaciens*
3B1	19	*D. cinnamea* *S. cohnii*	3B2	6	*S. epidermidis*

Source: Kroeger, B. (2017) STERIS Corporation.

The results of the *in situ* case study indicate the use of detergents as cleaning agents for residue removal and bioburden reduction is superior to WFI when heavy disinfectant residue is present. A formulated neutral detergent was more effective for these types of residues over a formulated oxidative detergent, however, a formulated oxidative detergent was as effective for residue removal when given a slightly longer contact time. WFI is recommended for routine use on a more frequent basis with detergents used on a monthly, quarterly, or biannual basis. The post-cleaning samples were taken prior to disinfection in this study. It is expected the bioburden would be significantly reduced after application of the disinfectant, thus it is recommended to follow the cleaning procedure with an application of disinfectant and sporicidal agent once the cleaning agent is rinsed or removed via mopping, wiping, or squeegee.

TABLE 7.3

Environmental monitoring sample results, prior to and post residue removal using sterile neutral detergent

Sterile neutral detergent					
Before Cleaning			After Cleaning		
EM Sample ID	Results cfu/plate	Microbial Isolates	EM Sample ID	Results cfu/plate	Microbial Isolates
1C1	10	*B. licheniformis*	1C2	9	*B. marisflavi*
2C1	19	*B. subtilis*	2C2	<1	N/A
3C1	7	*O. kimchi* *B. amyloliquefaciens*	3C2	9	*Sporosarcina soli*

Source: Kroeger, B. (2017) STERIS Corporation.

TABLE 7.4

Environmental monitoring sample control results prior to and post residue removal

Control – random sampling					
Before Cleaning			After Cleaning		
EM Sample ID	Results cfu/plate	Microbial Isolates	EM Sample ID	Results cfu/plate	Microbial Isolates
1D1	2	*M. luteus*	1D2	<1	N/A
2D1	4	*S. cohnii*	2D2	<1	N/A
3D1	10	*Bacillus (Solibacillus) isronensis*	3D2	2	*B. megaterium*

Source: Kroeger, B. (2017) STERIS Corporation.

7.9 BEST PRACTICES

The industry best practice in residue removal is to remove residues on cleanroom surfaces on a periodic basis based on visual observations of the residue build up and accumulation. Most cleanroom operations will remove residues either once a week, bi-weekly, monthly, or quarterly with a residue removal/rinsing step. The residue removal step typically involves WFI, 70% IPA, or a sterile cleaner for residue removal. A risk assessment should be performed to determine the frequency of cleaning based on the factors outlined in Figure 7.18. Start off less conservative and increase frequency based on visual observations

The objective of routine residue removal is to give the cleanroom surfaces a cleaner and more pristine image. Recent discussions with FDA regulators have indicated that excessive residues may signal to them that the cleanroom operation has

Environmental cleaning frequency
determined by:

- ISO Classification of area
- Activity in area or use
- Environmental monitoring
  feedback
- Type of process being
  performed, and equipment
  used
- Materials of construction
  in cleanroom
- Visual observations

FIGURE 7.18 Factors to consider for risk assessment used to determine cleaning frequency.

other issues as well and the residues may be hiding a bigger problem. Therefore, it is prudent and practical to periodically remove residues to prevent bigger issues from occurring in the cleanroom operation over time.

Cleaning/disinfection procedures should be written to ensure the operators can easily follow the procedure to avoid deviations in the procedure and ensure consistency and compliance. Best practice is to form a team of subject matter experts from each area, so their concerns are incorporated into the new procedure. There should not be multiple ways to clean areas of similar classifications unless they pose a higher risk as determined by a risk assessment. Even then, it should be easy to identify areas of higher risk such as Grade D areas adjacent to uncontrolled areas or Grade C areas adjacent to Grade A/B areas.

It is best practice to have a dedicated or specially trained team to perform facility cleaning/disinfection and avoid using janitorial companies to perform high-level cleaning and disinfection. It is imperative the personnel performing the facility cleaning and disinfection have specific training in cleanroom access and behaviors, microbial control, sterility assurance, personnel flow through the facility, and an understanding in disinfectant efficacy, use of sterilants, safe handling, and application techniques.

Most importantly, a rinse strategy should be included in site cleaning procedures to address how and when to rinse and to conduct a periodic cleaning without the use of a sanitizer, disinfectant or sporicide on a routine basis, to remove residues. Supplemental instructions should be included to underscore the importance of ensuring the surface is dry prior to disinfectant application, after a surface has been cleaned and rinsed, to avoid dilution of the disinfectant.

Consider the use of one product or a combination of products that are used throughout the facility instead of multiple product choices. Identify the circumstances, based on risk assessment, where one might be used over the other, eliminating any variability. A typical cleaning regimen in an aseptic processing area consists of application of a high-level cleaner disinfectant daily to walls, floors, and horizontal surfaces in

Grade A, B, and C areas and weekly in Grade C and D areas to floors and horizontal surfaces (walls may be cleaned monthly in D areas following a risk assessment), followed by a weekly (in a Grade C area) and monthly application of sporicidal agent in a Grade D area. Grade A/B areas require a sporicidal application pre-use. Use of a high-level disinfectant may be less routine or used during post-clean activities only. Residual disinfectant on stainless steel or glass may be removed with either ethanol, isopropyl alcohol, or WFI.

Disinfectant residue on floors and walls may be removed by a periodic deep cleaning monthly, quarterly, or as needed, using a sterile detergent such as a neutral cleaner. A routinely scheduled WFI rinse in a disinfectant program will help to limit or even prevent residue build up and thus avoid the requirement for a remedial clean. The frequency will be determined by disinfectant application frequency, however, residual disinfectant is typically rinsed after 30 applications prior to the application of the sterilant

Monitor residue build up and increase the frequency of rinsing if visible residue on the surface is appearing. The cleaner may be applied in a manner that is not in alignment with typical application of a disinfectant, i.e. using unidirectional, overlapping strokes. The objective of the cleaning step is to loosen soil on the surface so mechanical action is preferred using circular motion with approved cleaning utensils that are compatible with the cleaner. Cleaned surfaces are then rinsed using WFI. It is not required to rinse a high-level cleaner disinfectant after every application. The residue buildup in a month is minimal compared to the application of a cleaner.

Clean all tables, chairs, benches, desks, carts, and external surfaces of equipment by applying the cleaning agent to all surfaces using saturated wipes or sprayers. If the disinfectant/sanitizer is applied as a mist, wipe the surface as an auxiliary step to provide cleaning, if accessible.

It is acceptable to squeegee surfaces after disinfectant/sanitizer is applied using a saturated wipe or mist on glass or mirrored surfaces. Cleanroom curtains should be rinsed for visible residue removal after each application of disinfectant or sporicidal agents. Since these surfaces are difficult to clean due to their pliability, two people may be required where one individual holds the curtain while the other individual wipes the surface using a mop or saturated wipe, Figure 7.19. Alternatively,

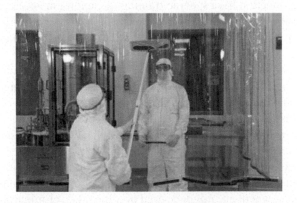

FIGURE 7.19 Technique for disinfectant application or residue removal from cleanroom curtains using two operators. Source: Kroeger, B. (2017) STERIS Corporation.

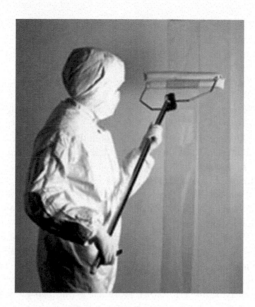

FIGURE 7.20   Micronova™ Curtain Cleaner™ handle. Source: Courtesy of Micronova™ (2018) www.micronova-mfg.com/products/hardware-accessories/curtain-cleaner-handle/Web.

cleanroom equipment specific to the task may be easier to use and only require one operator. Figure 7.20 is an image of a Micronova™ Curtain Cleaner™ handle that can clean both sides of the curtain at the same time.

7.10   CONCLUSION

Regular sanitization, disinfection, sporicidal use, rinsing, and periodic cleaning are all important aspects of the entire environmental control program as demonstrated by the examples given in this chapter. The frequency of each should be ascertained using a risk assessment based on factors such as classification, activity, substrates, environmental control, and visual criteria. Residue removal is an important part of this program since heavy residue can impact the integrity of the cleanroom and the equipment therein leading to efficacy concerns or deterioration, as noted in recent regulatory guidance documents. Having a program in place to control and mitigate residue build up in cleanroom environments can be considered an industry best practice. Lastly, consider not only residue contribution from the disinfection rotation program but also from manufacturing itself since residues may be introduced from any number of sources.

REFERENCES

1. Parenteral Drug Association (PDA) Technical Report # 70, Fundamentals of Cleaning and Disinfection Programs for Aseptic Manufacturing Facilities. October, 2015.
2. U.S. Food and Drug Administration, Inspections, Compliance, Enforcement, and Criminal Investigations, Compliance Actions and Activities, Inspectional Observation Summaries. www.fda.gov/ICECI/EnforcementActions/ucm531890.htm#Drugs. Accessed January 10, 2018.

3. PIC/S Guide to Good Practices for the Preparation of Medicinal Products in Healthcare Establishments. March 1, 2014.
4. Technical Regulation of Good Manufacturing of Drug Products, ANVISA Resolution-RDC n. 17, April 16, 2010.
5. United States Pharmacopeia (USP) 40, General Chapter <1072> Disinfectants and Antiseptics. 2018.
6. PDA Technical Report # 70, Fundamentals of Cleaning and Disinfection Programs for Aseptic Manufacturing Facilities (2015, October).
7. U.S. Food and Drug Administration, Inspections, Compliance, Enforcement, and Criminal Investigations, Ranier's Compounding Laboratory Warning Letter, March 28, 2017. www.fda.gov/iceci/enforcementactions/warningletters/2017/ucm558496.htm
8. Good Manufacturing Practice (GMP) Trends Issue # 974 GMP Trends LLC.P.O. Box 1111 Firestone, Colorado 80520 (August 15, 2017).
9. ASTM A380/A380M-17, Standard Practice for Cleaning, Descaling, and Passivation of Stainless Steel Parts, Equipment, and Systems. ASTM International, West Conshohocken, PA, 2017. DOI:10.1520/A0380_A0380M-17, www.astm.org.
10. Lopolito, P., Deal, A., and Klein, D. (2015) Strategies for Biofilm Remediation. *Cleanroom Technology* 22: 22–24.
11. FDA Inspections, Compliance, Enforcement, and Criminal Investigations, Warning Letter SEA 14-01, November 27, 2013. Available at: https://www.fda.gov/ICECI/Enfo rcementActions/WarningLetters/2013/ucm377891.htm
12. FDA Inspections, Compliance, Enforcement, and Criminal Investigations, Warning Letter 17-PHI-08, March 28, 2017. Available at: https://www.fda.gov/iceci/enforceme ntactions/warningletters/2017/ucm558496.htm
13. STERIS Technical Tip #4047, Recommendations for Drain Cleaning in Critical Environments.
14. Polarine, J. and Kroeger, B. (2016) How Issues Related to Utilities, Surfaces, and Practices Impact Cleanroom Environments. *Contamination Control in Healthcare Product Manufacturing, Volume 4*: 106–107.
15. Lopolito, P., Deal, A., and Klein, D. (2015) Strategies for Biofilm Remediation. Cleanroom Technology. 22: 22–24.
16. PDA Technical Report # 70, Fundamentals of Cleaning and Disinfection Programs for Aseptic Manufacturing Facilities (2015, October).
17. European Union (EU) GMP Annex I Manufacture of Sterile Medicinal Products, Draft 2018.

8 Microbiological Concerns in Non-Sterile Manufacturing

Jim Polarine, Jr. and Joe McCall

CONTENTS

8.1 INTRODUCTION

Virtually all pharmaceutical manufacturing is performed under non-sterile conditions. Even for sterile products (aseptically filled or terminally sterilized), the environment in which these products are manufactured and filled cannot be considered sterile. What is sterile? The scientific definition is the total absence of life. For pharmaceuticals, the definition for products labeled sterile is based on the probability of a single unit having viable microbial contaminants. The minimal acceptable standard is no more than one in 1,000,000 for terminally sterilized products, which can be qualified through scientific assessment of the sterilization process (e.g., gamma irradiation or saturated steam at high temperatures). For sterile products produced via aseptic processing with its countless sources of potential contamination, the probability of contamination is assessed through aseptic process simulations (media fills) where a minimal standard is no more than one in 10,000, although there is no actual way to calculate this number for aseptic processing. Risk and actual contaminated product are not synonymous terms. However, current technology will not support 100% sterility checks.

Pharmaceutical products, whether labeled as sterile or non-sterile, are always required to be safe for their intended purposes. The actual and potential microbial content are major factors in performing a product safety assessment. For manufacturers of sterile pharmaceuticals and biologic medical products produced by aseptic processing, there is a wealth of information in the form of regulatory guidance and requirements, standards, and industry literature that manufacturers can draw upon. For manufacturers of non-sterile products however, there seems to be a far lesser volume of available information, and it is less prescriptive than that which applies to sterile medicines. Given the relative scarcity of guidance and the array of product types and manufacturing processes, contamination control programs vary widely across the non-sterile industry. Federal guidance documents are rife with references to "appropriate", "reasonable", and "suitable" measures to assess and control contamination, but what is appropriate, reasonable, or suitable? One federal guidance calls for relevant operators to be "...free from abnormal sources of microbiological contamination (for example, sores and infected wounds)" [1] ... but what is "abnormal"? Are manufacturers compliant if they have a "no leprosy" policy? Far from it. The federal regulations and guidance documents stipulate only the most rudimentary and broadly defined standards. Why? Because they must be applicable across the wide swathe of all non-sterile manufacturers, encompassing every variant of product and process types in the industry. The federal regulations represent the minimum that manufacturers MUST adhere to. By no means does adherence to the minimum guarantee a safe and effective product. It is up to each manufacturer to understand the relevant characteristics of their own product and processes, and to deploy a scientifically sound contamination control program to ensure product and patient safety.

8.1.1 The Special Case of Non-Sterile Manufacturers

For manufacturers of sterile products produced by aseptic processing, any level of microbial contamination (in the product) is considered to wholly adulterate and render the product unfit for use. This concept is frequently, and speciously, extended to the controlled environments where these products are made. It is common for any level of microbial presence, when detected from environmental monitoring (EM) of the aseptic processing area's critical zone or support areas, to trigger an in-depth investigation that may ultimately result in rejection of the finished product. The consequent "shotgun" approach to contamination control, where the aim is to eliminate any and all microbial presence, can involve aggressive cleaning and chemical disinfection strategies, use of sterilized gowning, lengthy written procedures governing employees' aseptic behavior and techniques, and incorporation of complex (and expensive) equipment, utilities, and facility design – all earnestly deployed in the endeavor to keep microbial contamination out of the products and processes.

By contrast, the non-sterile manufacturer's contamination control program is typically less advanced, as some – but not all, microbial presence in the environment and the product itself is acceptable. In fact, without the aseptic processing "shotgun" approach to contamination control, it is entirely predictable and fully expected that there be some level of microbial presence in non-sterile manufacturing. The great challenge for non-sterile manufacturers is to determine what is a sufficient level of control, and how one discerns between microbial presence that is acceptable and that which puts the product at risk. The goal for non-sterile manufacturers is always to produce safe and effective medicines. This is especially challenging with the variety of factors that can introduce and influence microbial contamination in non-sterile manufacturing environments. Given these conditions, one could argue that the microbial contamination control programs for non-sterile manufacturers must be much more finely tuned and the staff in charge of these programs must possess a deeper level of understanding of pharmaceutical microbiology.

This chapter presents the principal microbiological considerations for manufacturers of non-sterile pharmaceuticals, with strategic information for non-sterile manufacturers to achieve contamination control programs that are risk-based, scientifically sound, and suitable for their specific products and processes.

How do products become contaminated with microorganisms? There is a very simple answer to this question and that is microorganisms entered or were incorporated into the product. What are potential sources of contaminants?

1. People
2. Raw materials and components
3. Equipment
4. Environment

In non-sterile products, the issue is not the potential for non-sterile units but rather what are acceptable levels of microorganisms in the product, and what types of microorganisms are not allowed. The pharmaceutical microbiologist has the task of assessing the amount and types of contaminants based on actual data and not theoretical risk. Most non-sterile products should and would fail a standard sterility test. There is not a requirement that they be free of microorganisms. Some non-sterile products whose base formulation will support microbial growth or survival may contain antimicrobial preservatives. These preservatives do not convey absolute contamination control however, in that there can be unaffected organisms and capacities that prevent complete control. The various preservative evaluation methods available (including the compendial methods) are designed to predict certain aspects of preservative performance. These methods are not fool-proof nor totally reliable [2].

The single paramount microbiological issue for non-sterile manufacturers is how to produce a safe product and the secondary aspect is what a safe product is. For the purposes of this chapter, the in-use issues around microbial contaminants and non-sterile products will only be briefly addressed. Manufacturers have very little practical control over consumer introduced contaminants. Products can be preserved, package design can limit contamination potential, and directions for use can include precautions and quantities of product limited to preclude extended use. However, manufacturers can rely on at least some portion of the consumers to do the unexpected. Unfortunately, manufacturers have been held liable on numerous occasions for product contaminated in-use by the consumer and causing some type of injury. Inadequate preservation has also been responsible for product recalls. This chapter concentrates on microbial contamination issues surrounding manufacturing operations when the manufacturer can have a reasonable opportunity to affect the finished product's microbial content.

It is not the intent or purpose of this chapter to quote regulations, guidelines, or standards. These are continuously developing as industry and science progress, so any such quotes would likely be outdated in a short period of time. Rather, established principles of contamination control coupled with a risk and science-based approach is presented. In other words, for non-sterile manufacturers, the importance of sound science surpasses a retelling of regulatory guidance and requirements.

8.1.2   What Is Sound Science?

Sound science is data derived from methods of proven capability.
Sound science uses facts not opinions or paradigms.
Sound science questions before acceptance.
Sound science looks for the truth regardless of the potential outcome.
Sound science is driven by logic, avoiding logical fallacies.
Sound science is data driven.

8.2   ORIGINS OF MICROBIAL CONTAMINANTS

Microbial contaminants can have diverse origins. The paradigm that Grade A/ISO 5 clean rooms are "sterile" contributes to the assumption that some significant error had to occur to result in a contaminated product. The several definitions of sterile add to the confusion and misunderstandings. The scientific definition of sterile is "without life". Processed foods use the term "commercial sterility" which loosely means that the product does not contain potentially harmful microorganisms. For aseptically filled or terminally sterilized pharmaceutical products, sterile refers to the likelihood of a contaminated single unit. A sterility test can have different meanings based on the culture or regulations. For example, in the United States, a sterility test is a specified procedure used to detect the absence of specific types of microorganisms in a volume of product. In other countries, a sterility test may also simply mean the determination of microbial content.

There is nothing abnormal or strange about finding microorganisms in a non-sterile environment. Consequently, finding microbial contaminants in products not labeled or rendered sterile should be expected and anticipated. As discussed in the chapter introduction, the possible sources of viable contaminants are not difficult to identify. The goal in non-sterile manufacturing should be to control, not eliminate, potential contaminants.

Viable contaminants are unique in that they can increase in level and occasionally be replaced or supplemented by other types of viable contaminants. A chemical contaminant may increase in quantity with time only if it is a break-down or degradation product of some formulation ingredient. That is to say there is a mass balance within the material in question. This approach does not apply to viable contaminants as the mass involved in even significant levels of microbial contaminants is relatively small. What may happen is that microorganisms can metabolize many different materials and leave metabolic by-products that can have significant adverse consequences for the product. Examples are pH shifts, color changes, odors, endotoxin and other toxins, and various enzymes. The first response to a suspected contamination problem should not be to discount it or assume it is a lab error of some type. This same misunderstanding frequently occurs when evaluating the potential for microbial contamination or the possible consequences of such an event. Spontaneous generation – life arising from non-life – was disproved in 1864 by Louis Pasteur. The fact that a contamination event occurred can only be refuted by another fact that it did not. The level of proof required for a scientific certainty is far greater than the legal requirement of "more likely than not".

8.3 EVALUATING THE POSSIBLE EFFECTS OF MICROBIAL CONTENT

The key issue concerning microbial contaminants in non-sterile products is the potential for those organisms to harm the user. If the product is protected from microbial contamination, degradation, or induced changes then the consumer will also be protected. Products can be involved in microbial-related adverse events in several ways. The manufacturer can partially control only certain aspects and those are the microbial content of the finished product and through antimicrobial preservatives the in-use microbial content. Primary package design such as non-aspirating applicators, single-use containers, single-use applicators also provide some protection. The manufacturer cannot prevent the consumer from intentionally or inadvertently contaminating the product by trying to dilute it, mixing it with other products, storing it under adverse conditions, sharing it with others, or using it contrary-to-label directions.

8.4 MICROBIAL GROWTH AND CHARACTERISTICS

Before the potential effects of microbial contaminants can be evaluated, the presence of contaminants, their concentration, and their identity must be determined. Microorganisms do not exist in nature as pure cultures. The use of pure cultures was developed to better study the characteristics of specific organisms. In nature, microorganisms often exist in biofilms which are composed of multiple species each contributing to the evolution and survival of the biofilm structure. These biofilms can shed organisms into the surrounding environment at varying rates or be disrupted by mechanical or chemical means resulting in a massive release of organisms. A biofilm can contain many different environments which are inhabited by organisms specific to that environment. It is imperative that manufacturers employ pharmaceutical microbiologists with the appropriate education and sufficient level of experience in order to assess the risks that microbial contaminants pose to patient safety and product quality.

8.5   DETECTION METHODS AND CAPABILITIES

The methods used to detect the presence and quantities of microorganisms are many and varied. However, none are totally reliable or capable of detecting all organisms. A method is composed of several components including sampling, sample holding, sample transport, sample processing, and culturing. Each separate component or activity has multiple potential variables. The expectations and assumptions about method capabilities and their ability to provide accurate, reliable information has resulted in specifications and limits that are often unrealistic. The United States Pharmacopeia (USP) acknowledges at least 50% variability in the standard plate count procedure and states that a material or product with an APC (aerobic plate count) limit of 100 cfu (colony forming units) should not be considered out-of-specification unless the test shows 200 cfu [3]. The methods used to demonstrate method suitability acknowledge the inability of the methods to quantitatively recover organisms directly from the material or product tested. The suitability methods require that test organisms be quantitatively recovered from a dilution of the product or material, not the actual product or material. The antimicrobial preservative efficacy test (APE) necessitates the recovery of organisms from the actual preserved product [4]. However, it is not usually possible to recover the complete test inoculum immediately after inoculation in most products. Objective evaluations of commonly used methods have shown time after time that the expectations of that method, as shown by specifications referencing the method, are not within the capability of the method. For example, one should not presume there is a meaningful difference between the detection of one cfu or five cfu from a surface monitored by contact plates.

Microorganisms exist in many shapes, sizes, and configurations; they can be spherical (cocci), rod-shaped (bacilli), helical, or any variety of forms in between (see Figure 8.1, coccobacilli shape, in between a sphere and a rod). Their nutritional state and growth conditions can affect all these characteristics, many times unpredictably. Conventional detection methodology and attendant specifications assume

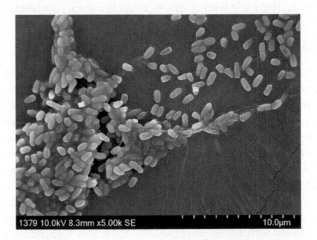

FIGURE 8.1   Pseudomonas aeruginosa 5,000X magnification inside silicone tubing Special thanks to Stacey Gish and Bruce Ritts at STERIS Corporation for the SEM image in Figure 1.

that these factors are a constant. In establishing specifications, the assumption is made that a colony forming unit (cfu) is synonymous with a single organism even though the term cfu was coined to acknowledge the fact that this was not the case for most species of microorganisms. In fact, a single colony may have indeed arisen from a single progenitor cell, or it may have initially arisen from a thousand or more microbial cells. Visual observation of one singular colony cannot convey, with absolute certainty, that it came from one singular bacterial cell. This fact more than any other shows the fallacy of establishing specifications based on the number of recovered organisms using conventional cultivation-based test methodology. The term conventional refers to the classic culture techniques where the organisms must grow to be detected either by forming a visible colony, measurable change in their environment, or visible evidence of their presence. Newer, unconventional methodologies include gene probes, antigen, measuring ATP, ADP, DNA, or RNA levels, and other such parameters. The basic science and the first use of these unconventional methodologies goes back many years. Advances in instrumentation and the drive for more sophisticated and thus presumed better, faster methods have pushed the development and use of such alternative techniques.

8.6 EVALUATING RECOVERED ORGANISMS

When microorganisms are recovered from a product or material those organisms should be evaluated for significance, relative to the nature of the recovered organism and the product's intended use (i.e. route of administration, patient population, etc.). The presence of microbial contaminants in products purported to be sterile renders those products unfit for use. However, products not labeled as sterile require a different approach.

> Where warranted, a risk-based assessment of the relevant factors is conducted by personnel with specialized training in microbiology and the interpretation of microbiological data. For raw materials, the assessment takes account of processing to which the product is subjected, the current technology of testing and the availability of materials of the desired quality. [3]

8.7 HOW TO PERFORM A RISK ASSESSMENT
USING COMPENDIAL GUIDANCE

There are many factors that comprise a risk assessment for a non-sterile commercial product. Various guidance documents exist but there is no assurance that complying with guidance document requirements or suggestions will assure a risk-free product. A microbiological risk assessment is an informed judgment about the potential for any microbial contaminants to cause harm to a user. This assessment should be conducted by "personnel with specialized training in microbiology and the interpretation of microbiological data" [3].

In the simplest and most basic terms, the presence of viable (and sometimes nonviable) microorganisms poses a risk of those organisms causing an infection or some type of toxic reaction for the user. Even sterile products present a risk, particularly after first use. The environments in which we all live contain numerous different types and species of microorganisms. The fact that most of these organisms do not cause obvious or overt harm demonstrates that certain conditions must exist before the mere presence of viable microorganisms is a cause for concern. The expectations of most consumers are that products they buy, and use should be safe for their intended purposes. Manufacturers do not produce and sell products that they know pose an unreasonable risk of causing harm. The purpose of a risk assessment is to determine, from the facts available, if the product would pose an unreasonable risk if used as intended. The label directions should specify the intended method of use. A manufacturer may wish to consider the potential effect on safety if a consumer were to use the product in a foreseeable but contrary-to-label directions manner. For example, it is reasonable to predict that some consumers may drink directly out of a bottle when the use of a spoon was specified on the label; the risks inherent to this misuse should be considered by the manufacturer.

In conducting a risk assessment, the first evaluation should be the potential for the product to support microbial growth or survival. If microorganisms can proliferate within the product, then the potential for harm is greatly increased over a product that will only allow survival but not growth. Unless a product is naturally inhibitory to microbial growth or survival (for example has pH extremes, low water activity, or antimicrobial components), the presence and efficacy of specifically added antimicrobial preservatives must be considered. Antimicrobial preservatives can have one of three effects on contaminating microorganisms:

1. No effect
2. Retard growth
3. Kill

What effect, if any, is very dependent on the type of organism, the quantity, storage conditions, other formulation components and time. Whether a preservative system retains efficacy over time must be considered as well as what organisms will naturally challenge that system either during manufacturing and storage or use. The manufacturer has far more control over conditions and potential microbial content during manufacturing than during use. If any specific types or species of organism are known safety issues with the specific or similar products, then these should be specifically evaluated for potential to cause harm in connection with the specific product being assessed. The various evaluation methods for preservative efficacy do not require the complete kill of challenge organisms even after 28 days.

Once the actual and potential microbial content of the product has been assessed, then that information can be used in further assessments based on the remaining compendial criteria. The identity to genus and species of any organisms in a product subsequent to manufacture but prior to distribution needs to be determined. However, frequent name changes with time and improved identification methods make literature searches to the species level and many times even to the genus level problematic. Consequently, assessments need to be made using probabilities based on Gram reaction, colonial morphology, microscopic appearance, etc. as well as various identification methods. For example, Gram-positive spore-forming rods capable of aerobic growth only have certain species that would normally be considered pathogenic for humans. The majority of Gram-negative organisms are opportunistic pathogens and a large number are human pathogens [5].

An organism capable of causing a disease is referred to as a pathogen. An organism that will cause a disease or set up an infection under certain circumstances is called an opportunistic pathogen. The relative ability of any organism to cause a disease or set up an infection is called virulence. Those characteristics of the organism or condition of the host that facilitate an infection are called virulence factors. Certain microbial disease processes are caused by the organism itself or by some metabolic byproduct of that organism. Humans as well as other animals harbor many different types and species of microorganisms that are necessary for the body's proper function. This is called a commensal or symbiotic relationship. When these organisms migrate from their "normal" body location to other locations they can and will cause an infection. Other organisms that would be considered normal micro flora can undergo genetic changes or be replaced by a different strain of the same species and become pathogenic. A weed has been described as a plant that is growing in the wrong place. This analogy can be made for resident micro flora. The point of this review is that any microorganism is an unknown regarding its ability to cause harm. The factors that can and should be considered when evaluating the virulence of organisms in a product are:

- the use of the product: hazard varies according to the route of administration (eye, nose, respiratory tract);
- the method of application;
- the intended recipient: risk may differ for neonates, infants, and the debilitated;
- use of immunosuppressive agents, corticosteroids;
- presence of disease, wounds, organ damage.

8.8 THE USE OF THE PRODUCT: HAZARD VARIES ACCORDING TO THE ROUTE OF ADMINISTRATION (EYE, NOSE, RESPIRATORY TRACT)

The ability of any microbial contaminant to cause harm is directly related to its ability to colonize/grow on/infect the host. The body has certain non-specific defense mechanisms against infection including natural barriers such as the skin, lysozyme in tears, low pH in the intestinal tract, amebocytes and interferon in the circulating blood, mucous and hair to trap and filter organisms in the nose, etc. Consequently, the route of administration can and will affect the potential of organisms to infect the user. The eye provides a significant barrier unless the cornea is scratched. Such scratching can occur with contact lenses, fingernails, dirt, inadvertent injuries, etc. The eye has very little vascularization meaning that any type of defense depending on circulation will be hindered. The respiratory tract and intestinal tract provide routes where the skin barrier is bypassed. The low pH in the intestinal tract protects against many organisms. However, the respiratory tract provides only limited natural host defenses. Consequently, inhaled product such as nasal sprays can put the user at increased risk.

8.9   THE METHOD OF APPLICATION

Leave-on as opposed to apply-and-remove products provide longer potential contact times. Aerosols or sprays provide more potential surface area contact and possibility of inhalation. Reusable applicators are higher risk than one-time applicators. Diluting a product for use often dilutes the antimicrobial preservative system below useful levels. Any type product that is designed to be injected or used on broken or abraded skin is a great risk because it bypasses the skin barrier.

8.10   THE INTENDED RECIPIENT: RISK MAY DIFFER FOR NEONATES, INFANTS, AND THE DEBILITATED

The common factor here is that any natural host defenses may be compromised either because they are not fully developed (neonates/infants) or have deteriorated based on age or physical condition. Regardless of the root cause, the potential increased risk of infection is the same. Other than labeling, the manufacturer has very little if any real control over the potential users of their products. However, if it is conceivable that such individuals could use the product, the potential to cause risk for the user should be considered.

8.11   USE OF IMMUNOSUPPRESSIVE AGENTS, CORTICOSTEROIDS

These types of drugs will reduce the effectiveness of host defenses against infection. The ability of the manufacturers to restrict use of their product by such individuals is limited to labeling.

8.12   PRESENCE OF DISEASE, WOUNDS, ORGAN DAMAGE

These conditions will make a potential user more susceptible to infection through several mechanisms. Again, the manufacturer may intend their product for such individuals or may want to restrict use via labeling. A manufacturer who designs a product for use by diseased and debilitated people needs to consider the potential consequences of any microbial contaminants.

Taking the above considerations into account, it is still very difficult to make the judgment call to release a product containing viable non-pathogenic organisms or which has a propensity to become contaminated during usual and customary use. The manufacturer assumes the risk for potential harm to the user. The manufacturer must decide if the non-prescription product is unreasonably dangerous, as unlike prescription products there is no one else, such as a physician or pharmacist, to inform or counsel the potential user.

8.13   MICROBIOLOGICAL CONTROL

In products labeled sterile, microbiological control is achieved in two ways. The first and most reliable is terminal sterilization. The second method is aseptic manufacture. The regulatory standards for each method reflect the differences in controllability.

Regardless of method, the manufacturer must develop systems and procedures to control the bioburden of the product. In non-sterile products, the presence of viable organisms must be expected. A balance must be struck between the degree of control (including cost) and the needed level of control. Risk can be mitigated by controlling the formulation and the manufacturing environment. The sources of potential contaminants are easily identified:

1. People
2. Raw materials and other components
3. Equipment
4. Environment

8.14 PEOPLE

It is well known that the number one source of contamination in pharmaceutical manufacturing is people. It is equally well known that terminal sterilization would be an effective control measure but is not practical. Consequently, other measures must be used. Official guidelines and regulations specify minimum control measures which primarily consist of "bagging" the workers and training them in various methods to minimize breaching the "bag" or coming in contact with external contaminants and exposing the product to those contaminants. Variations of this approach range from "clean" uniforms to fully enclosed and pressurized suits that are externally sterilized.

Normal human skin is colonized with bacteria; different areas of the body have varied total aerobic bacterial counts (e.g., 1×10^6 colony forming units (CFUs)/cm^2 on the scalp, 5×10^5 CFUs/cm^2 in the axilla, 4×10^4 CFUs/cm^2 on the abdomen, and 1×10^4 CFUs/cm^2 on the forearm). Total bacterial counts on the hands of medical personnel have ranged from 3.9×10^4 to 4.6×10^6. The issues with people are confining the inherent contaminants to prevent spread and controlling behavior so that fomites will not be a source of contamination [6].

8.15 RAW MATERIALS AND OTHER COMPONENTS

These represent a major control point for product contamination. Unless raw materials and primary packaging components are sterilized or the finished product sterilized, the bioburden of these items must be considered. A heat step in the process or a filtration step or some other part of the process can reduce the bioburden. However, reliability requires that such steps be clearly stated to be bioburden reducing and that the appropriate controls and effectiveness evaluations must be included. Particularly in raw materials and to a certain extent bulk and finished product the assumption cannot be made that microbial contamination is or will be uniform. Patterns of contamination are a topic unto themselves. It is sufficient at this point to state that contamination should be expected to be randomly distributed, non-uniform, and of variable levels in non-sterile materials that will support microbial growth or survival. Sampling plans should be designed with such variability in mind. A common mistake made in designing sampling plans and sampling methods to detect bioburden is to assume the only concern is the bulk material and not areas of likely contamination. For example, sampling below the top surface, sampling the center of drums or bags only risk missing likely points of contamination. Materials that are hydroscopic will exhibit higher moisture levels on top or side surfaces. Airborne contaminants will more likely be on the top surface or bottom of bags and drums because containers are many times left open prior to filling and prior to closing after filling. Unless there is a policy of discarding the top and bottom material, the total contents will be included in the manufacture of the finished product.

8.16   EQUIPMENT

Equipment including primary contact and incidental contact can and will be a source of microbial contaminants. The ideal situation would be for all primary contact equipment to be sterilized. This is not possible in many situations. One alternative is to use disposable, sterile liners but these are not without cost. Even sterilized or sanitized equipment can be a problem based on storage conditions and the presence of low level residuals. Condensate can be a major potential problem. A 500 L tank with 1 ml of condensate that contained 50,000,000 CFUs (5×10^{-7}) would start with 100 CFUs per ml of product.

As previously discussed, microbial contaminants can and will increase in level under the proper conditions. Even the use of antimicrobial preservatives may not prevent or mitigate this problem. The best control measure is to sanitize the equipment immediately before use and to keep hold times to a minimum. Hot water rinse (60° C) has been shown to be a very effective control measure in numerous applications. Sanitizing conditions are generally acknowledged to be 60° C for ten minutes with shorter exposure times using higher temperatures. Blocks of metal such as pump housings can act as heat sinks and require more exposure time to reach temperature.

8.17   ENVIRONMENT

Environmental conditions including air borne organisms, general sanitation level of the facility, and similar concerns can have a real or presumed adverse effect on the product being manufactured in the area. Proving an effect or no-effect is not an activity that would be value-added in many situations. It is better to defer to the paradigm that says contaminated areas lead to contaminated product, i.e. the higher the level of ambient contamination, the greater the chance of a contaminated product. So, every reasonable effort should be made to minimize area contamination and the opportunity to expose product to contamination. Simple precautions include a cleaning sanitization program, physical barriers such as shields and doors that stay closed, use of gloves and appropriate uniforms, air flow patterns, etc. A monitoring program is useful but should be designed with the type and end use of the product in mind. For example, in manufacturing a non-sterile powder for topical use, the ability of microorganisms to survive or reproduce in such products is minimal when compared to water-based liquid. Extensive environmental controls and monitoring aimed at controlling potential microbial contamination would be of little value to product safety in such a situation.

REFERENCES

1. U.S. Food and Drug Administration, Code of Federal Regulations Title 21 Vol.2, Part 117, Subpart B – CGMP Sec. 117.10 Personnel (a), www.accessdata.fda.gov/scripts/cdrh/cfdocs/cfCFR/CFRSearch.cfm?CFRPart=117&showFR = 1&subpartNode = 21:2.0.1.1.16.2, 2017.
2. Farrington, J. K., et al., Ability of laboratory methods to predict in-use efficacy of antimicrobial preservatives in an experimental cosmetic. *Applied and Environmental Microbiology*, 60: 4553–4558, 1994.
3. United States Pharmacopeia (USP) 41 < 1111> Microbiological examination of non-sterile products: Acceptance criteria for pharmaceutical preparations and substances for pharmaceutical use. HYPERLINK "http://app.uspnf.com/uspnf/" http://app.uspnf.com/uspnf/ access 09/06/2018.
4. USP 41 <51> Antimicrobial Effectiveness Testing. http://app.uspnf.com/uspnf/ access 09/06/2018.
5. Bergey, D. H., Noel R. Krieg, and John G. Holt. *Bergey's Manual of Systematic Bacteriology*. Baltimore, MD: Williams & Wilkins, 1984.
6. Selwyn, S., Microbiology and Ecology of Human Skin. *Practitioner*, 224: 1059–1062, 1980.

9 Preservatives and Why They Are Useful

Jeanne Moldenhauer

CONTENTS

9.1 INTRODUCTION

Preservatives are utilized in a variety of products (e.g., pharmaceutical formulations, cosmetics, and foods) in order to control the microbial bioburden of the product. There are a variety of preservative properties that are commonly desired across product types: the ability to have broad spectrum effectivity against microbial organisms (both Gram-positive and Gram-negative microorganisms and fungi); are chemically stable over the product's shelf life; they are non-toxic or have low toxicity; they are not adsorbed by the container; are compatible with other additives in the formulation; and should not be affected by changes in pH. When selecting a preservative, it is important to understand how the product is intended to be used (Anonymous, 2017a). Other common considerations when selecting and using preservatives include: ease of use, solubility for liquid products, and cost.

It can also be beneficial to combine more than one type of preservative in a formulation. Some of the benefits include: may have a wider range of activity; reduced toxicity; reduced incidence of resistance; and the potential to be used in lower concentrations. Propylene glycol is often added to emulsion products that have parabens in order to reduce loss due to micelles (Anonymous, 2017a).

9.2 WHAT IS A PRESERVATIVE?

It is a common practice to add chemical substances to parenteral formulations for a variety of different reasons. These include: antioxidants, buffers, bulking agents, chelating agents, antimicrobial agents, solubilizing agents, surfactants, and tonicity-adjusting agents. The purpose of these additives is to ensure that the final product is safe, efficacious, and meets the product specifications (Avis et al., 1992).

Some of the pharmacopeias have specifications for the type and amount of additives that may be added to products – dependent upon the route of administration. Typically, this is not harmonized across compendia, so it is important to understand the intended markets for products to ensure that you understand all of the applicable requirements (Avis et al., 1992).

According to the U.S. Library of Medicine (2017) a preservative (pharmaceutical) is defined as: "Substances added to pharmaceutical preparations to protect them from chemical change or microbial action. They include ANTI-BACTERIAL AGENTS and antioxidants" (emphasis original).

However, pharmaceuticals are not the only products that utilize preservatives. Preservatives are widely used in foods, cosmetics, some medical devices (e.g., some ophthalmic products), and pharmaceuticals. Typically, the products are used routinely and require a long shelf life. Frequently these products have a high water content that could lead to degradation if a preservative is not used (Anonymous, 2017b).

Preservatives are required for multiple-dose pharmaceutical products unless specifically prohibited by the monograph or unless the drug itself is bacteriostatic or bactericidal. They may be added to individual unit-dose containers which are not terminally sterilized. The preservatives may be considered an adjunct to aseptic processing – being able to eliminate low levels of contamination that may have occurred during the aseptic process (Avis et al., 1992).

Some products are specifically prohibited from having preservatives or anti-microbial agents, like large-volume parenterals which are provided to supply fluids, nutrients, or electrolytes (Avis et al., 1992).

9.3 CLASSIFICATION OF PRESERVATIVES

There are a variety of different methods that can be used to classify preservatives.

9.3.1 CLASSIFICATION OF PRESERVATIVES BASED UPON THE MODE OF ACTION

9.3.1.1 Antioxidants

This category of preservatives prevents oxidation of the active ingredient and is used in the case where the active pharmaceutical ingredient degrades by means of oxidation (they are sensitive to oxygen) (Shaikh et al., 2016).

Table 9.1 provides information on some examples of antioxidants.

9.3.1.2 Antimicrobial Agents

These chemicals are effective against microorganisms that can cause product degradation.

Table 9.2 provides examples of antimicrobial agents.

TABLE 9.1
Examples of Antioxidants

Antioxidant	Maximum Concentration used in Parenterals (%)	Source of Information
Acetone sodium bisulfite	0.2	Avis et al., 1992
Ascorbic acid	0.01	Avis et al., 1992
Ascorbic acid esters	0.015	Avid et al., 1992
Butylhydroxyanisole (BHA)	0.02	Avis et al., 1992; Shaikh et al., 2016
Butylhydroxytoluene (BHT)	0.02	Avis et al., 1992; Shaikh et al., 2016
Cysteine	0.5	Avis et al., 1992
Glutatathione	0.1	Avis et al., 1992
Nordihydroguairetic acid (NDGA)	0.01	Avis et al., 1992
Monothioglycerol	0.5	Avis et al., 1992
Sodium bisulfite	0.15	Avis et al., 1992
Sodium metabisulfite	0.2	Avis et al., 1992
Tocopherols	0.5	Avis et al., 1992
Vitamin C	Not Stated	Shaikh et al., 2016
Vitamin E	Not Stated	Shaikh et al., 2016

TABLE 9.2
Examples of Antimicrobial Agents

Antimicrobial Agent	Maximum Concentration used in Parenterals (%)	Source of Information
Benzalkonium chloride	0.01	Avis et al., 1992
Benzelhonium chloride	0.01	Avis et al., 1992
Benzyl alcohol	1–2	Avis et al., 1992
Butyl ρ-hydroxybenzoate	0.015	Avis et al., 1992
Chlorobutanol	0.25–0.5	Avis et al., 1992
Chlorocresol	0.1–0.3	Avis et al., 1992
Metacresol	0.1–0.3	Avis et al., 1992
Methyl ρ-hydroxybenzoate	0.18	Avis et al., 1992
Nitrates	Not Stated	Shaikh et al., 2016
Phenol	o.5	Avis et al., 1992
Phenylmercuric nitrate and acetate	0.5	Avise et al., 1992
Propyl ρ-hydroxybenzoate	0.2	Avis et al., 1992
Sodium benzoate	Not Stated	Shaikh et al., 2016
Sorbates	Not Stated	Shaikh et al., 2016
Thimerosol	0.01	Avis et al., 1992

9.3.1.3 Chelating Agents

These substances prevent degradation by the formation of complexes with the active ingredient.

Table 9.3 provides examples of these types of agents.

9.3.2 CLASSIFICATION OF PRESERVATIVES BASED UPON THE PRESERVATIVE SOURCE

Preservatives can be obtained from a variety of sources, e.g., natural or artificial.

TABLE 9.3
Examples of Chelating Agents

Chelating Agent	Maximum Concentration used in Parenterals (%)	Source of Information
Citric acid	Not Stated	Shaikh et al., 2016
Disodium ethylenediaminetetraacetic acid (EDTA)	Not Stated	Shaikh et al., 2016
Ethylenediaminetetratraacetic acid salts	0.01–0.075	Avis et al., 1992
Polyphosphates	Not Stated	Shaikh et al., 2016

9.3.2.1 Natural Preservatives

This classification refers to preservatives that are obtained from natural sources like plants, minerals, and the like. Some examples include: diatomaceous earth, honey, lemon, neem oil, sodium chloride (salt), sugar, and vinegar (Shaikh et al., 2016).

In the food industry, some common processes may be used to achieve preservation, e.g., freezing, pickling, salting, and smoking. Some preservatives target enzymes in fruits and vegetables, which can metabolize even after cutting. Some examples include: citric acid and ascorbic acid form lemonor. Citrus juice inhibits the action of phenolase, which turns apples and potatoes brown when they are cut open Shaikh et al., 2016).

9.3.2.2 Artificial Preservatives

This classification refers to preservatives that are man-made, usually by chemical synthesis and are active against low levels of microorganism. Some examples include: benzoates, nitrites, propionates, and sodium benzoate sorbates (Shaikh et al., 2016).

9.4 CHOOSING THE RIGHT PRESERVATIVE

There are a number of considerations that must be made in selecting the appropriate preservative to utilize in your process, including for example: route of administration of the product, compatibility of the preservative with the product formulation, the effects of the preservative on product stability, and so forth.

9.4.1 COMMON PRESERVATIVES AND ROUTE OF ADMINISTRATION

Table 9.4 identifies some of the common preservatives and which ones are used with different routes of administration of the product.

9.4.2 ORAL SUSPENSIONS AND ISSUES WITH PRESERVATIVE EFFECTIVENESS

Selecting a preservative also involves maintaining the activity of the preservative in the product. To do this properly, one needs to select the correct form of the preservative, the right concentration to ensure that microbial proliferation is inhibited, and an understanding of other factors that may affect efficacy of the preservative. Some of these concerns include: the formulation pH, the presence of micelles, and the presence of hydrophilic polymers (Anonymous, 2017a).

9.4.2.1 Formulation pH

For some products, it can pose a problem to use an acidic preservative like benzoic acid or sorbic acid. The preservative, in its active form may be ionized or unionized. For example, benzoic acid is undissociated in the active form. The pKa of benzoic acid is 4.2, meaning that it is active at a pH below 4.2, where it remains in the unionized form. This form is able to diffuse across the outer membrane of the microorganism and over time into the cytoplasm. The preservative dissociates in the cytoplasm due to the neutral conditions present. This results in acidification of the cytoplasm and inhibition of growth (Anonymous, 2017a).

TABLE 9.4

Examples of Common Preservatives Used in Specific Routes of Product Administration

Route of Product Administration	Preservative	Chemical Class of Preservative	pH of Optimum Activity	Source of Information
Oral	Methyl, ethyl propyl polyparapens and combinations	Amino aryl acid esters		Elder and Crowley, 2012
	Sodium benzoate, benzoic acid	Aryl acids	Aryl acids pH <4.5	Elder and Crowley, 2012; Elder and Crowley, 2017
	Sorbic acid, potassium sorbate, propionic acid	Alkyl acids	Alkyl acids pH 3.9 Sorbic acid pH 4.5	Elder and Crowley, 2012; Elder and Crowley, 2017
	Methyl paraben and sodium benzoate combination	Amino aryl acid esters/ organic acid		Elder and Crowley, 2012
	Butyl paraben (concentration 0.006–0.05% oral suspension)	Not stated		Anonymous, 2017a
Topical including nasal products	Benzalkonium chloride, cetrimonium bromide, benzelthonium chloride, alkyltrimethylammonium bromide	Quaternary ammonia compounds (QACs)	QACs pH 4–10 pH 7–9 Benzylthonium chloride pH 4–10	Elder and Crowley, 2012; Elder and Crowley, 2017
	QACs, e.g., benzalkonium chloride, EDTA	QACs and metal chelator	QACs pH 4–10	Elder and Crowley, 2012; Elder and Crowley, 2017
	Methyl, ethyl, propyl, butyl parabens and combinations butyl parabens (concentration 0.02–0.4% topical formulation)	Amino aryl acid esters	Aminoben-zoate esters (parabens) pH 4–8	Elder and Crowley, 2012; Elder and Crowley, 2017; Anonymous, 2017a

(Continued)

TABLE 9.4 (CONTINUED)

Examples of Common Preservatives Used in Specific Routes of Product Administration

Route of Product Administration	Preservative	Chemical Class of Preservative	pH of Optimum Activity	Source of Information
	Benzyl alcohol, cetyl alcohol, steryl alcohol	Alkyl/aryl alcohols	Aryl alcohols pH <5	Elder and Crowley, 2012; Elder and Crowley, 2017
	Benzoic acid, sorbice acid	Alkyl and aryl acids (salts)	Aryl acids pH <4.5; Alkyl acids pH 3.9	Elder and Crowley, 2012; Elder and Crowley, 2017
	Chloroactamide, trichlorocarban	Alkyl and aryl amides		Elder and Crowley, 2012
	Thimerosal	Organomercurials	Thimerosal pH 5–8	Elder and Crowley, 2012; Elder and Crowley, 2017
	Imidurea, bronopol	Formaldehyde donators	Formaldehyde donators pH 3–9	Elder and Crowley, 2012; Elder and Crowley, 2017
	Chlorhexidines	Biguanides	Biguanides pH 5–7	Elder and Crowley, 2012; Elder and Crowley, 2017
	4-Chlorocresol, 4-chloroxylenol, dichlorophene, hexachlorophene	Phenols	Chlorocre-sol pH 4–7; Phenols pH 4–9	Elder and Crowley, 2012; Elder and Crowley, 2017
Parenterals (including vaccines)	Benzyl alcohol, chlorbutanol, 2-ethoxyethanol	Alkyl/aryl alcohols	Aryl alcohols pH <5	Elder and Crowley, 2012; Elder and Crowley, 2017
	Methyl, ethyl, propyl, butyl parabens and combinations	Amino aryl acid esters	Aminoben-zoate esters (Parabens) pH 4–8	Elder and Crowley, 2012; Elder and Crowley, 2017
	Benzoic acid, sorbic acid	Alkyl/aryl acids	Aryl acids pH <4.5	Elder and Crowley, 2012
	Chlorhexidene	Biguanides	Biguanides pH 5–7	Elder and Crowley, 2012; Elder and Crowley, 2017

(Continued)

TABLE 9.4 (CONTINUED)

Examples of Common Preservatives Used in Specific Routes of Product Administration

Route of Product Administration	Preservative	Chemical Class of Preservative	pH of Optimum Activity	Source of Information
	Phenol, 3-cresol	Phenols	Phenols pH 4–9	Elder and Crowley, 2012
	Thimerisal, phenylmercurate salts	Organic mercurials	Thimerisal pH 5–8	Elder and Crowley, 2012; Elder and Crowley, 2017
Ophthalmic	QACs e.g., benzalkonium chloride (and others)	QACs	QACs pH 4–10 pH 7–9 Benzalkonium chloride pH 4–10	Elder and Crowley, 2012; Elder and Crowley, 2017
	QACs/EDTA	QACs/metal chelator	QACs pH 4–10 pH 7–9	Elder and Crowley, 2012; Elder and Crowley, 2017
	Themerosal, phenylmercurate salts	Organic mercurial		Elder and Crowley, 2012 Anonymous, 2017a
	Phenylethyl alcohol, phenoxetol and benzalkonium chloride are combined and used in eye drops.	Not stated		
	Benzoic acid, sodium benzoate, sorbic acid, potassium sorbate	Alkyl/aryl acids	Aryl acids pH <4.5 Alkyl acids pH 3.9	Elder and Crowley, 2012; Elder and Crowley, 2017
	Chlorhexidine, polyaminopropylbiguanide	Biguanides	Biguanides pH 5–7	Elder and Crowley, 2012 Elder and Crowley, 2017
	Imidurea	Formaldehyde donators	Formaldehyde donators pH 3–9	Elder and Crowley, 2012; Elder and Crowley, 2017

9.4.2.2   Micelles

Preservatives that have lipophilic properties (e.g., the unionized form of acidic preservatives, phenolics and parabens), can result in the partitioning of these formulations into micelles. When this happens, the concentration of available preservative in solution is reduced (Anonymous, 2017a).

9.4.2.3   Hydrophilic Polymers

If there are hydrophilic polymers present in oral solutions, like polyvinylpyrrolidone, and methylcellulose, the free concentration of preservative in the product formulation is reduced. This is a result of the preservative's ability to chemically interact with the dissolved polymer. One way to address this is to increase the concentration of preservative in the product formulation, if possible. Sometimes, the preservative may be incompatible with hydrophilic polymers due to electrostatic interaction. As such, it is inappropriate to use cationic hydrophilic polymers with acidic preservatives in oral solution products (Anonymous, 2017a).

9.4.2.4   Use of Plastic Containers

When integral glass containers are utilized, it is expected that the preservative (antimicrobial) effectiveness is maintained. If plastics are utilized, additional care must be used in selecting the preservative. With a plastic container, it is possible for the preservative to permeate through the container or have adsorption of the preservatives into the internal plastic surface. The use of cationic antimicrobial agents may be limited, due to the positive charge of the preservative may change the surface charge of drug particles. Additionally, they may be incompatible with a number of adjuvants (Anonymous, 2017a).

9.4.2.5   Factors That Can Result in Loss of Preservative Action

There are several common situations that may result in the loss of preservative action including: solubility in oil, interaction with emulsifying agents and suspending agents, interactions with the container, and volatility.

9.4.3   Preservative Modes of Action

In general, preservatives are not effective against viral contamination. Some may be bactericidal and fungicidal. They may act on several different microbial cellular targets, e.g., the cell wall, the cytoplasmic membrane or the cytoplasm. You may not be able to identify the specific target for the preservative. The target can change based upon the preservative concentration. Some examples of the ways that preservatives can interfere with microbial cellular mechanisms is provided in Table 9.5 (Elder and Crowley, 2012).

9.4.3.1   Preservatives Affecting the Cell Wall

This affect may be due to the lysis as a result of enzyme inhibition, e.g., with the phenols and organo mercurials. However, glutaraldehyde's effect is due to irreversible cross-linking at the cell wall (Elder and Crowley, 2012).

9.4.3.2 Preservatives Affecting the Cytoplasmic Membrane

It is believed that this effect may be a result of effects on the membrane potential, membrane enzymatic function or a generalized membrane permeability. The preservatives cetrimide, chlorhexidine, hexachlorophene, 2-penoxyethanol, parabens, and phenols all affect the membrane permeability. They allow the "leaking" of essential cell constituents that in turn results in the cell dying. Sorbic acid works to inhibit the transport mechanisms across the cytoplasmic membrane and suppressed fumarate oxidation. The preservative chlorhexidine inhibits the enzyme ATPase. This results in the inhibition of cellular anaerobic activity. If the preservative concentrations are elevated it causes the precipitation of cytoplasmic nucleic acids and related proteins. The biguanide preservatives cause phase separation and the formation of domains in the phospholipid bi-layer. The chelating agents like edetic acid (EDTA) affect the cytoplasmic membranes integrity as it chelates the divalent calcium and magnesium ions, and thus the ions are unavailable to the microbial cell and other antimicrobial agents. The quaternary ammonium compounds used as preservatives bind strongly to the cytoplasmic membrane resulting in general damage to the membrane and subsequent leaking. They particularly target the phospholipid bi-layer (Elder and Crowley, 2012).

9.4.3.3 Preservatives Affecting the Cytoplasm

The cytoplasm may be affected by the uncoupling of the oxidative and phosphorylation processes or by interference with the active transport mechanisms. This is how weak carboxylic acid and alcohol-based preservatives work. Some preservatives inhibit the electron transport chains, which results in inhibition of metabolic activity in aerobic bacteria. The preservatives benzoic acid and the parabens inhibit the synthesis of folic acid. The bronopol and organo mercurial preservatives target thiol enzymes that are present in the cytoplasm. The formaldehyde donators like imidurea act on the carboxylic and amino enzymes in the cytoplasm. The phenols and alcohols work by causing protein denaturation (Elder and Crowley, 2012).

9.5 REGULATORY EXPECTATIONS FOR USE OF PRESERVATIVES

There are several regulatory expectations for the use of preservatives in a product formulation. They include: proof of efficacy, safety information, control mechanisms in the finished products, and labeling details for the finished product. The way the preservatives work can also be different as shown in Table 9.5.

9.5.1 PERFORMANCE EXPECTATIONS FOR PRESERVATIVES

If preservatives are used in the formulation, it is important to assess whether the preservative accomplishes the desired characteristic. Some of the typical characteristics that may be desired from the preservative include: antimicrobial activity, aqueous solubility, partitioning behavior, stability, non-irritant, organoleptic properties, and compatibility (Elder and Crowley, 2012).

TABLE 9.5
Preservatives Microbial Targets

Preservatives Affecting the Cell Wall	Preservatives Affecting the Cytoplasmic Membrane	Preservatives Affecting the Cytoplasm
Phenols	2-Phenoxyethanol	2-Phenoxyethanol and other organic alcohols
Aryl and alkyl acids	Parabens	Aryl and alkyl acids
Organo mercurials	Organo mercurials	Halogenated preservatives
EDTA (edetic acid)	EDTA	
Chlorhexidine, cetrimide	Chlorhexidine, hexachlorophene	Chlorhexidine (high concentrations)
Glutaraldehyde	Formaldehyde donators, e.g., bronopol, imidurea	Formaldehyde donators, e.g., bronopol, imidurea
Anionic surfactants	Benzylkonium chloride (BKC)	

Source: Adapted from Elder and Crowley, 2012.

TABLE 9.6
Preservative Performance Characteristics and Methods to Assess Effectiveness

Desired Characteristic	Method to Assess Effectiveness
Antimicrobial activity	Effective against bacteria and fungi at low levels of contamination.
Aqueous solubility	Solubility exceeds the minimum inhibitory concentrations (MIC) over the anticipated pH range of the product.
Partitioning behavior	Remains consistently in the aqueous phase in multiphase products.
Stability properties	Chemically and physically stable over the product shelf life.
Non-irritant properties	Non-irritating at the concentration used. This is very important for products used on mucosal tissues, e.g., eyes, ears, and nose.
Organoleptic properties	Odor and taste are acceptable for oral dosage forms, intranasal dosage forms and for inhalation forms. The last two of these dosage forms have a portion of the medication that is swallowed.
Compatibility	Does not react adversely with the product formulation or the container – closure system. If there is any reaction, it is minimal.

Source: Adapted from Elder and Crowley, 2012.

Table 9.6 provides various preservative characteristics and methods to assess the efficacy of the preservative in meeting the desired characteristic.

9.5.2 Preservative Effectiveness Testing (PET) AKA AntiMicrobial Effectiveness Testing (AET)

The pharmacopeias for the United States (USP, 2010), Europe (EP, 2010), and Japan (JP, 2010) all have requirements to show that the products manufactured do not support the growth of microorganisms if exposed to microbial contamination and that if contamination is present, it will be reduced to acceptable levels. This test requirement is called either the preservative effectiveness test (PET) or the anti-microbial effectiveness test (AET) (Snowdon, 2012).

This testing involves the use of defined microorganisms to challenge the abil-ity of the product's preservative ability to keep contamination at an acceptable level. Within the test method, one inoculates a specified number of organisms along with environmental isolates from your site, and then evaluates the level of growth present over time up to 29 days. The test organisms harmonized from all pharmacopeia include: *Staphylococcus aureus, Pseudomonas aeruginosa, Aspergillus niger* (Aka *Aspergillus brasiliensis),* and *Candida albicans.* Both United States Pharmacopeia (USP, 2010) and Pharm Europa (EP, 2010) also indi-cate that *Escherichia coli* should be used. In some cases, there are specific organ-isms of concern for a specific facility or process. Some regulators expect that these organisms are also tested. A major organism of concern these days, espe-cially for non-sterile, aqueous-based products is *Burkholderia cepacia,* which is an opportunistic pathogen (Elder and Crowley, 2012). It is also recommended to utilize some environmental isolates in this testing to ensure that the types of con-tamination seen at your size and whether it will be affected by your preservation system.

The acceptance criteria for the USP (2010) and JP (2010) are predominantly simi-lar. However, there are some differences between product type and presentation. All of the compendia have similar requirements for the reduction of the challenge organ-isms with no subsequent increase from the initial count after 14 and 28 days. It is important to note that the Pharm Europa (EP, 2010) is considered the more stringent and challenging requirement to meet. In this case, there is a specified reduction in bacterial count within the final 14 days, and no subsequent increase from the initial count after 14 and 28 days (Elder and Crowley, 2012).

Table 9.7 compares the requirements of the USP and EP for antimicrobial effec-tiveness testing of bacteria.

Table 9.8 compares the requirements of the USP and EP for antimicrobial effec-tiveness testing of fungi (yeasts and molds).

It is important to perform these studies as part of the initial validation of the preservative system. Additionally, the preservative effectiveness must be confirmed during stability at the end of product shelf life. Some regulatory agencies may require that additional studies are performed during the use life, especially if the container is opened and closed repeatedly (Elder and Crowley, 2012).

Rapid microbiological methods (RMMs) have been evaluated as possible replace-ments for the compendial test method. Some RMMs are able to provide actual organ-ism counts, while others have different reporting units, e.g., relative light units. Some of the methods that do not use organism counts may still be validated for use, as they can easily detect whether there is a difference in recovery and/or detect no growth being present. Generally, RMMs are qualified using EP 5.1.6 (2010) or USP < 1223> (2010). Depending upon the regulatory authority a prior approval supplement may be required prior to implementation.

TABLE 9.7

Comparison of USP and EP Requirements for Antimicrobial Effectiveness Testing Total Viable Bacteria

Pharmacopeia	Time Points Bacterial Log Reductions						
	6 hrs.	24 hrs.	2 days	7 days	14 days	21 days	28 days
USP Category 1				<1.0	<3.0		No increase from 14-day count
USP Category 2					<2.0		No increase from 14-day count
USP Category 3					<1.0		No increase from 14-day count
USP Category 4					No increase from initial count		No increase from 14-day count
EP Category A1 (Suggested)	<3.0	No recovery	No recovery	No increase	No recovery	No recovery	No recovery
EP Category B2 (Minimum)		<1.0		<3.0			No increase

Source: Elder and Crowley, 2012.

TABLE 9.8

Comparison of USP and EP Requirements for Antimicrobial Effectiveness Testing Total Viable Fungi (Yeasts and Molds)

Pharmacopeia	Time Points Fungal Log Reductions							
	6 hrs.	24 hrs.	2 days	7 days	14 days	21 days	28 days
USP Category 1				No increase from initial count	No increase from initial count	No increase from initial count	No increase from 14-day count
USP Category 2					No increase from initial count	No increase from initial count	No increase from 14-day count
USP Category 3					No increase from initial count	No increase from initial count	No increase from 14-day count
USP Category 4					No increase from initial count	No increase from initial count	No increase from 14-day count
EP Category A1 (Suggested)			<2.0		No increase	No increase	No recovery
EP Category B2 (Minimum)					<1.0	No increase	No increase

Source: Elder and Crowley, 2012.

9.6 PRODUCTS WITHOUT PRESERVATIVES

Some manufacturers promote their products as being superior due to the lack of preservatives, e.g., food and cosmetics. This can lead to expectations from users that pharmaceuticals would be better without preservatives. While, some formulations can be safely made without preservatives, at this time preservatives are required for some products like multiple-use containers. If preservatives are not present, the supplier must show that microorganisms cannot grow in these products (Elder and Crowley, 2012).

However, if there is a regulatory requirement to have a preservative, e.g., a multi-use sterile pharmaceutical product, if you choose not to use a preservative, it is expected that you will perform the antimicrobial effectiveness test anyway to show that the product itself provides the microbial safety level required.

In fact, in recent years many sterile and non-sterile products have been required to show that microorganisms cannot grow in the product, due to the time period associated with administration of the product and/or the time period prior to administration after breaching the container-closure system. Metcalfe (2009) This testing method is similar to a preservative effectiveness test, even though no preservative is present. This test method is dependent upon the product's ability to prevent growth of the microorganism over the typical use time (times two or three)

9.7 TYPICAL CONSIDERATIONS/CONCERNS WITH USE OF PRESERVATIVES

Several questions were proposed and answered by Snowdon (2017) regarding the use of preservatives. Some of these questions are repeated here, with abbreviated answers.

9.7.1 IS THE ADDITION OF A KNOWN PRESERVATIVE SUFFICIENT TO CONTROL CONTAMINATION?

When selecting the appropriate preservative system, one still needs to understand the potential for interactions with the product formulation or the container-closure system. Another consideration is the expected activity of the preservative against different microorganisms (Snowdon, 2012).

9.7.2 IS PACKAGING A CONCERN WITH PRESERVATIVE USE?

The packaging material can play a part in issues with the preservative, e.g., leaching into the packaging can lower preservative levels. As such, changes in packaging materials should necessitate studies on the preservative's effectiveness (Snowdon, 2012).

9.7.3 DOES THE STORAGE CONDITIONS AFFECT PRESERVATIVES?

Some microorganisms do not proliferate at low temperatures. Others are not inhibited by refrigeration. As such, it is possible to have unintended metabolites (Snowdon, 2012). It is common to find fungal contamination routinely in low temperature storage devices.

9.8 CONCLUSION

Maintaining the microbiological quality of your products is critical. Preservatives can play a vital role in the ability to prevent contamination of your products. Failure to add preservatives can cause issues for your products during their shelf life. However, care must be taken in selection of the appropriate preservative system to use. Once an initial decision is made on the preservative choice, validation testing must be conducted in accordance with the appropriate compendia to ensure that the preservative system is efficacious.

LITERATURE CITED

Anonymous (2017a) Preservatives Used in Pharmaceutical Suspensions. Downloaded from: http://formulation.vinensia.com/2011/12/preservatives-used-in-pharmaceutical.html on September 14, 2017.

Anonymous (2017b) Pharmaceutical Preservatives, Preservative Suppliers in India. Downloaded from: http://preservativesindia.com/preservative-manufacturers.htm on October 17, 2017

Avis, K. E., Lieberman, H. A., and Lachman, L. (1992) *Pharmaceutical Dosage Forms: Parenteral Medications Volume 1*, 2nd Edition, Revised and Expanded. Marcek Dekker, Inc., New York. Chapter 5: Formulation of Small Volume Parenterals, (DeLuca, P. P. and Boylan, J. C.) pp. 173–248.

Elder, D. P. and Crowley, P. J. (2012) Antimicrobial Preservatives Part One: Choosing a Preservative System. *American Pharmaceutical Review*. Downloaded from: www.a mericanpharmaceuticalreview.com/Featured-Articles/38886-Antimicrobial-Preservati ves-Part-One-Choosing-a-Preservative-System/on September 14, 2017. Note: the print copy of this article was in the July-August, 2017 issue.

Elder, D. P. and Crowley, P. J. (2017) Antimicrobial Preservatives Part Two: Choosing a Preservative. *American Pharmaceutical Review.* Downloaded from: www.americanpha rmaceuticalreview.com/Featured-Articles/343543-Antimicrobial-Preservatives-Part-Two-Choosing-a-Preservative/ on October 25, 2017.

European Pharmacopoeia (EP) (2010) 5.1.3 Efficacy of Antimicrobial Preservation, EP 6.4. European Directorate for Quality of Medicines, Strasbourg, France.

Japanese Pharmacopeia (JP) (2010), General Information: 19. Preservative Effectiveness Test, 15th Edition. Society of Japanese Pharmacopeia, Tokyo, Japan.

Metcalfe, J. W. (2009) Microbiological Quality of Drug Products After Penetration of the Container System for Dose Preparation Prior to Patient Administration. Downloaded from: www.americanpharmaceuticalreview.com/1429-AuthorProfile/2530-John-W-Me tcalfe-Ph-D/ on October 24, 2017.

Shaikh, S. M., et al. (2016) A Review on: Preservatives used in Pharmaceuticals and impacts on Health. *PharmaTutor*, 4(5): 25–34.

Snowdon, G. (2012) Preventing Contamination with Preservatives. *PharmTech.com.* Downloaded from: www.pharmtech.com/preventing-contamination-preservatives on October 17, 2017.

United States Pharmacopeia (USP) (2010) General Chapter < 51 > Antimicrobial Effectiveness Testing, USP 34-NF29. Rockville, MD.

U.S. Library of Medicine (2017) Definition of Preservative, Pharmaceutical. Downloaded from: www.definitions.net/definition/preservatives,%20pharmaceutical on October 17, 2017.

10 The Problem of *Burkholderia cepacia* Complex (BCC) in Your Facility

Jeanne Moldenhauer

CONTENTS

10.1 WHAT IS BCC?

BCC is an abbreviation of *Burkholderia cepacia* complex. Microbewiki defines this term as, "*Burkholderia cepacia* complex is a group of Gram-negative, non-spore-forming bacilli that are composed of approximately 17 closely-related species which are grouped into nine genomovars" (Microbewiki, 2017). Another definition says, "Burkholderia cepacia complex, or simply *Burkholderia cepacia*, is a group of catalase-producing, lactose-nonfermenting, Gram-negative bacteria composed of at least 20 different species, including *B. cepacia, B. multivorans, B. cenocepacia, B. vietnamiensis, B. stabilis, B. ambifaria, B. dolosa, B. anthina, B. pyrrocinia* and *B. ubonensis. B. cepacia* is an opportunistic human pathogen that most often causes pneumonia in immunocompromised individuals with underlying lung disease. Patients with sickle-cell haemoglobinopathies are also at risk. The species also attacks young onion and tobacco plants, as well as displaying a remarkable ability to digest oil" (Wikipedia, 2017).

"BCC can survive or multiply in a variety of non-sterile and water-based products because it is resistant to certain preservatives and antimicrobial agents," the US Food and Drugs Administration (FDA) said in a statement. "Detecting BCC bacteria is also a challenge and requires validated testing methods that take into consideration the unique characteristics of different BCC strains."

According to FDA, people exposed to BCC are at an increased risk for illness or infection, especially patients with compromised immune systems (FDA, 2017).

Another issue is that in the various reclassifications of microorganisms in recent years, many contamination risks in the past may have been called by other genus names, e.g., *Pseudomonas, Ralstonia,* and the like. As such, looking for historical information on these contaminants may be difficult.

Recently, there have been several articles and discussions on the regulatory interest in *B. cepacia* being identified in pharmaceutical facilities. (Torbeck et al., 2011) There are at least 18 different species of this organism, and several related organisms. Collectively they are referred to as BCC. The typical source of these organisms is water, although some have been found in soil, with prolonged survival in moist environments, and in biofilm formation (Ensor, 2017).

This organism is an opportunistic pathogen, and is associated with endocarditis, wound infections, IV bacteremia, foot infections, and respiratory infections. As such, this organism is a concern for aqueous products. It tends to show a resistance/persistence for organic solvents, antiseptics, disinfectants, and low nutrient states. It has also shown resistance to efflux pumps (Ensor, 2017).

It is important to note that there are also organisms closely related to BCC, which are not part of the official 20 species identified in BCC. One such organism is *Wautersia sp.* While not part of BCC, it causes similar issues to patients, is waterborne, and is hard to detect. Some identification systems may indicate that is has a low level probability of being BCC.

Originally, it was believed that this was only a concern for patients with cystic fibrosis or other immune-compromised individuals. However, in the 2016 time period, numerous "healthy" personnel were affected by the presence of *Burkholderia cepacia* in non-sterile products.

The US Centers for Disease Control and Prevention (CDC) claims that the bacteria is known to be resistant to many common antibiotics, making infection more difficult to treat (Mezher, 2016).

The FDA's current expectation is for companies to be aware of their concerns with BCC and to take immediate and comprehensive action to rid the facility of this contaminant. Additionally, companies must have product release tests to show the absence of *Burkholderia cepacia* for non-sterile aqueous products (FDA, 2017).

10.2 REGULATORY REQUIREMENTS FOR BCC TESTING

In 2017, FDA presenters indicated that BCC is a significant issue to the agency and identified that a new regulatory guidance was being prepared to address these concerns. This guidance was issued later in 2017 (Ensor, 2017; FDA, 2017).

10.2.1 HISTORY OF REGULATORY RECALLS DUE TO BCC

In 2016 and 2017 there were a variety of product recalls that were mandated by either FDA or the affected companies. All of these recalls were due to BCC. BCC contamination is believed to be due to water-borne contamination with opportunistic pathogens (Brennan, 2017). The following is a partial listing of the recalls that took place (Brennan, 2017):

- October 2016, an FDA investigation identified BCC in more than ten lots of oral liquid docusate sodium produced by Florida-based contract manufacturer PharmaTech. The recalled products include multiple lots of docusate sodium laxatives, cough syrup, antihistamines, and sodium citrate-citric acid, which is used to treat reduce urine acidity for patients with gout and kidney stones. However, PharmaTech says it has not received any reports indicating contamination in the additional products listed in the expanded recall. (Mezher, 2016,) This company found the contaminant in its water system. PharmaTech participated in a voluntarily recalled all its liquid products from 20 October 2015 through 15 July 2016 as a precautionary measure (Brennan, 2017).
- The US Centers for Disease Control and Prevention (CDC) identified 60 cases of BCC infection in eight states (Mezher, 2016).
- August 2016, Sage Products issued a recall notice for one lot of its Comfort Shield Barrier Cream Cloths, which treat and prevent moisture associated skin irritation, because of BCC contamination. (Brennan, 2017)
- A prescription, non-sterile nasal spray was found to be contaminated with *Burkholderia multivorans* another member of the *Burkholderia cepacia* complex (Ensor, 2017).

10.2.2 What Is Expected of Drug Manufacturers

The FDA has issued guidance in support of the requirements stated in the *Code of Federal Regulations* (FDA, 2017).

The following includes regulatory expectations for drug manufacturers (Brennan, 2017; FDA, 2017):

- "Establish procedures designed to prevent objectionable microorganism contamination of non-sterile drug products, such as procedures to assure adequate quality of incoming materials, sanitary design, maintenance and cleaning of equipment, production and storage time limitations, and monitoring of environmental conditions (21 CFR 211.113(a)).
- Use scientifically sound and appropriate acceptance criteria (e.g., USP Chapter < 1111 > Microbiological Examination of Non-sterile Products: Acceptance Criteria for Pharmaceutical Preparations and Substances for Pharmaceutical Use)8 and test procedures (e.g., USP < 61>/<62 > Microbiological Examination of Non-sterile Products: Microbial Enumeration Tests and Tests for Specified Microorganisms, respectively) to assure that drug product components (including pharmaceutical water) and finished drug products conform to appropriate quality standards (21 CFR 211.160(b)).
- Provide appropriate drug product specifications (tests, methods, and acceptance criteria) in applications submitted to the FDA (21 CFR 314.50(d)(1) for new drug applications, or 21 CFR 314.94(a)(9) for abbreviated new drug applications). As appropriate, additional laboratory tests may be needed to determine whether products are suitable for release.
- Ensure that the methods used to test finished drug products prior to release for distribution are appropriately validated, accurate, sensitive, specific and reproducible (21 CFR 211.165).
- Test in-process materials during the production process (e.g., at commencement or completion of significant phases, or after storage for long periods), using valid in-process specifications to ensure, e.g., that the drug product will meet its final specification, including criteria for absence of microbial contamination, where appropriate (21 CFR 211.110).
- Investigate any failure to meet specifications, including other batches of the same drug product and other drug products that may have been associated with the specific failure or discrepancy (21 CFR 211.192), and implement appropriate corrective and follow-up actions to prevent recurrence."

10.3 CONTROLLING THE MICROBIOLOGICAL QUALITY OF YOUR PRODUCTS

10.3.1 Understanding the Risk to the Patient

Important considerations for drug manufacturers include the quality attribute of patient risk. This attribute is affected by the drug products' route of administration, patient population, dosage form/formulation, the risk factors included in USP < 1111>, and the acceptance criteria for the product (Ensor, 2017).

10.3.1.1   Route of Administration

There are differences in the route of administration that may affect the severity of patient risk associated with the contamination of the product. Typical routes of administration include for example, gastrointestinal, mucosal, dermal, (transdermal patches with microneedles), inhalation, and the like. More detail is provided in USP < 1111> (Ensor, 2017).

Each of these areas of the body have different normal flora associated with them, and therefore different microorganisms may have different impacts depending upon where it is located. Some of the key environmental factors include: pH and mucous membranes (Ensor, 2017).

10.3.1.2   Patient Population

The risk of certain types of contamination vary based upon the patients that receive the medicine. Among patient populations, it is important to consider the elderly, infants, and immunocompromised individuals as they may be more significantly affected than healthy individuals (Ensor, 2017).

10.3.1.3   Dosage Form/Product Formulation

The type of dosage form plays a key role in microbiological quality. Some formulations may be bacteriostatic or bactericidal. The formulation is also affected by whether it is aqueous or non-aqueous, oil, or emulsion. In dry powders, the amount of water activity present plays a key role in whether microorganisms will proliferate in the formulation. Typically, a solid drug formulation which has a low water activity level (a_w). Non-solid, aqueous and non-aqueous formulations are differentiated by the level of water activity. In general, a water activity level of < 0.6 is considered non-aqueous. The lower the A_w level, the lower the microbiological risk associated with the product (Ensor, 2017).

10.4   SOURCES OF MICROORGANISMS IN PHARMACEUTICAL MANUFACTURING

Three major sources of contamination are possible: raw materials, the manufacturing process, and the manufacturing environment (Ensor, 2017).

10.4.1   RAW MATERIALS

Water is a key ingredient in many different pharmaceutical formulations. When present, water is a significant potential source of contamination to the product. As such, monitoring data should be available to ensure that any contamination present is controlled.

What are the sources of your raw materials, e.g., plant or animals? Animal sources have the potential for more types of contamination. How is the process controlled? Are the compendial excipients controlled to be within the USP limits for microbial limits testing? Is the total aerobic count and the total yeast and mold counts controlled within the compendial requirements? Additional information can be found in USP < 1111> (Ensor, 2017).

10.4.2 Manufacturing Process

One of the major concerns of the manufacturing process, is whether there are steps that are likely to have a potential for microbial proliferation. Do components of the formulation provide the opportunities for microorganism growth? Do hold times allow for proliferation? Are you doing a good job on housekeeping? Failure to properly clean could also add to the risk of contamination.

Microorganisms need food, water, and time to proliferate. If it is not possible to control the food and water, controlling the time at these conditions becomes critical. Keep in mind that even if a finished product has a very low water activity, extended aqueous hold steps may lead to microbial proliferation. As such, it is important to limit hold times and have performed testing to qualify the allowable hold times (Ensor, 2017).

USP < 1115>, Bioburden Control of Non-Sterile Drug Substances and Products, provides recommendations and references for a risk-based approach to establish a microbiological control program (Ensor, 2017).

It is important to minimize the risk of microbial contamination that might potentially cause: drug product degradation, introduction of microbial metabolites and/or toxins, and high levels of microorganisms, which may be critical depending upon the patient population (Ensor, 2017).

10.4.3 Manufacturing Environment

A major contributor to potential contamination is the personnel working in the process. Are there specific gowning procedures used in the process? Are the procedures followed? Are they effective?

Companies need to be compliant with the current good manufacturing practices for their operation. This includes having an effective system for cleaning, environmental monitoring, and compliant and controlled water systems (Ensor, 2017).

10.5 MICROBIOLOGICAL CONTROL MECHANISMS

There are widely accepted test methods and acceptance criteria for drug products in the compendial, e.g., USP < 61 > Microbial Enumeration Tests, USP < 62 > Tests for Specified Organisms, and the Total Aerobic Microbial Counts and the Total Combined Yeast and Mold Counts. The acceptance criteria for specific microorganisms are specified in USP < 1111>, Microbiological Examination of Non-Sterile Products Acceptance Criteria for Pharmaceutical Preparations and Substances for Pharmaceutical Use. USP < 1112 > describes the methods to apply water activity determination in assessing microbial risk to non-sterile products (Ensor, 2017).

Another mechanism that can be used is ICH Q6A, Test Procedures and Acceptance Criteria for New Drug Substances and New Drug Products: Chemical Substances. This document provides (Ensor, 2017):

- Recommendations for conditions which may allow for "periodic" or "skip testing" of microbial enumeration tests
- Upstream controls

- Component bioburden controls
- Low product A_w
- Manufacturing history
- Typically, solid oral dosage forms

10.5.1 AQUEOUS AND MULTI-DOSE PRODUCTS

Products that are aqueous and multi-dose must include an antimicrobial preservative or be self-preserving to prevent contamination. This methodology is specified in USP < 51 > the Antimicrobial Effectiveness Testing.

10.5.2 *BURKHOLDERIA CEPACIA* COMPLEX (BCC)

Opposition to this concern has been voiced by Sutton and Moldenhauer (Moldenhauer, 2012) believing that this organism was only a concern to high risk patients with cerebral palsy. However, in 2016, there was an outbreak of BCC drug incidents in dicoto liquid (docusate sodium liquid) that affected hospitalized patients with 13 deaths, 58 cases and 43 suspect cases. It affected at least eight states in the USA. The manufacturer of this product initiated a voluntary recall in May 2016 (Ensor, 2017).

Another incident happened with a normal saline flush (12 mL IV flush syringe with a 3 mL, 5 mL, or 10 mL fill). These syringes were recalled as a Class 1 device recall (Ensor, 2017).

Comfort Shield Barrier Cloths (2% chlorhexidine gluconate wipes) were also subjected to a voluntary recall, although no adverse events reported (Ensor, 2017).

A prescription, non-sterile nasal spray was found to be contaminated with *Burkholderia multivorans* another member of the BCC (Ensor, 2017).

These concerns have led regulators to develop a recommendation for BCC in aqueous, non-sterile drug products. This recommendation includes that the company provide a BCC risk mitigation strategy including a test method and acceptance criteria to demonstrate the drug product is free from BCC. They would also like to see a validation of this test method (Ensor, 2017).

The FDA has an impending publication for microbiological control of non-sterile drugs (Ensor, 2017).

10.6 CASE STUDIES WITH BCC

There have been several instances of BCC or believed BCC contamination with which the author has been personally involved. This section describes some of those circumstances and the corrective actions taken.

10.6.1 ORAL MOUTHWASH PRODUCTS

A pharmaceutical company manufactures a non-alcohol-based mouthwash One lot of this product, was recalled due to the presence of *Burkholderia cepacia* in the product. Another lot of the same mouthwash product was also manufactured. This lot tested negative for the *Burkholderia cepacia*, however it did show the presence of *Cupriavidus pauculus*. The contaminant was present and detected at 4 cfu/mL.

The release criterion at the pharmaceutical company for this product is "no objectionable organisms" as opposed to a criterion of "absence of Gram-negative organisms." A health risk assessment was conducted to evaluate the risks associated with this microorganism.

10.6.1.1   Background on the Organism *Cupriavidus pauculus*

Cupriavidus pauculus is a type of Gram-negative, non-fermentative, motile bacterium. It is from the genus of *Cupriavidus* and the family of *Burkholderiaceae*. It has been isolated from water, the water in hospital ultrafiltration systems, as well as bottled mineral water (Aspinall and Graham, 1989; Balada-Llasat et al., 2010; Clark et al., 1998; Ori et al., 1998; Manara et al., 1990; Anderson et al., 1997).

The organism isolated from the product was found to be Gram-negative, catalase, oxidase, citrate, and urea positive. It tested negative for indole, nitrate, methyl red-Voges-Proskauer, gelatin, and esculin. No acid production was found from glucose, xylose, mannitol, lactose, sucrose, or maltose. Triple sugar iron and litmus milk were alkaline, and motility was observed. It is described as *"Pseudomonas-like"* non-fermenting bacilli by some identification systems (Balada-Llasat et al., 2010).

The taxonomy of *Cupriavidus pauculus* is described below (UniProt Consortium, 2013; LPSN 2013):

Taxonomy Identifier	82633
Scientific Name	*Cupriavidus pauculus*
Synonym	*Ralstonia paucula, Wautersia paucula*
Other Names	ATCC 700817
	CCUG 12507
	CDC E6793
	CDC group IVc-2
	CIP 105943
Rank	Species
Lineage	– Cellular organisms
	– Bacteria
	– Proteobacteria
	– Betaproteobacteria
	– Burkholderiales
	– Cupriavidus
See also	NCBI

Over the years, there have been many instances of reclassification of the microorganisms in *Bergey's Manual*. In the case of this microorganism, it was previously classified as *Ralstonia paucula* (Vandamme et al., 1999) and *Wautersia paucula* (Vaneechoutte et al., 2004). As such, in investigating health risks, reports for both of these microorganisms also need to be considered.

Ralstonia paucula is described as a Gram-negative environmental bacterium. It is reported to be found in pool water, ground water, bottled mineral water, and clinical specimens. While it is not frequently found in clinical setting, it is recognized as an opportunist pathogen that is able to generate serious infections like septicemia, peritonitis, abscesses, and the like. These effects are more severe in immune-compromised patients (MicroWiki, 2013). This organism was also associated with serious nosocomial infections (Moissenet et al., 2001).

Ralstonia spp. has been implicated in various cystic fibrosis patients. One of the difficulties in the analysis is that it is difficult to differentiate between species of *Ralstonia*. Within this analysis of *Ralstonia*, they also include *B. cepacia* (Coenye et al., 2002).

Vandamme et al. (1999) describes *Wautersia paucula* as being identical to the *Ralstonia paucula*.

10.6.1.2 Health Risks Associated with *Cuprividus pauculus* (*Ralstonia paucula* and *Wautersia paucula*)

Cuprividus pauculus is rarely found as a pathogenic organism in humans, however when found it can cause significant disease especially in immune-compromised patients (Balada-Llasat et al., 2010). There are case reports of bacteremia, septicemia, peritonitis, abscess, and tenosynovitis. The source of the organism was not identified for all cases, but contaminated water was identified as the source in some patients. It has also been associated with nosocomial infections (Balada-Llasat et al., 2010).

However, Balada-Llasat et al. (2010) reported several case studies where the patients were exposed to the organism through the use of culturette swabs and contaminated tap water. None of these patients were immune-compromised yet they were not sure about the real pathogenicity of the organisms since they did not grow upon re-culture (after the initial isolation and identification) (Balada-Llasat et al., 2010).

Tasbakan et al. (2010) reported 19 cases of peritonitis and one case of tenosynovitis associated with *Cupriavidus pauculus*. For one of the cases the patient developed ventilator-associated pneumonia due to the *Cupriavidus pauculus* (Tasbakan et al., 2010).

Stovall et al. (2010) reported the nosocomial transmission of *Cupriavidus pauculus* during extracorporeal membrane oxygenation (ECMO). This was reportedly the first known case of infection using ECMO.

Cupriavidus pauculus has also been isolated as the causative agent in airway infections of individuals with cystic fibrosis (Kalka-Moli et al., 2009).

Unfortunately, since this organism is not routinely isolated as a pathogen in clinical settings, no data could be found identifying the concentration of microorganism that is required to cause a pathogenic action.

10.6.1.3 Conclusion of the Investigation

There are few reported cases of pathogenicity due to *Cupriavidus pauculus*, however when reported the infections caused by this organism can be severe. This reaction is worse in patients that are immunocompromised. Additionally, this organism has been found to be present in patient airways of those who have cystic fibrosis. While the drug company manufactures a mouthwash product, there is concern with the ability to transmit this organism as the reports have indicated it to be present in bottled mineral water (which would be most like the administration through mouthwash). None of the published articles have shown specific pathogenicity due to the contaminated mineral water in patients. Nor do any of the articles published provide information on the ability of a count of four colony forming units (cfu) to cause a pathogenic effect.

However, since this organism is hard to differentiate from other similar organisms and in many cases the publications listed in this report either had the identification testing performed at the *Burkholderia cepacia* Research Laboratory (recognized worldwide as experts in BCC) and/or performed the testing including *Burkholderia cepacia* in the test panel, there is a concern as to whether the identification is correct or whether there is a possibility that this is actually *Burkholderia cepacia*. This is further complicated by another recent lot of product being contaminated with *Burkholderia cepacia*. Like *Burkholderia cepacia* this organism has been shown to have significant health concerns to individuals with cystic fibrosis.

With no published information on the level of contamination necessary to trigger an infection, the concerns with the identification, and the knowledge that this is a water-borne organism (with water being the base diluent of the product), this organism was treated as objectionable to the product.

10.6.2   AQUEOUS NON-STERILE PRODUCTS

Because of the various recalls and concerns by other manufacturers regarding the presence of BCC in their facilities several different companies identified in their facilities. This case study is a compilation of several different investigations that were all treated and resolved in the same manner.

10.6.2.1   Health Concerns with This Organism

Based upon the various publications and presentations by FDA, it was well known that the presence of BCC was a significant health risk.

10.6.2.2   Changes to Manufacturing Practices during the Investigation

A common problem in non-sterile drug manufacturing is that environmental monitoring is performed at a much lower frequency than in sterile drug manufacturing facilities. Additionally, when contamination is found it is not typical to routinely identify every contamination event. As contaminated product was found, it was difficult to use the routine monitoring data to ensure that this organism was or was not present in the facility. Since the data was not reliable for use in this way, it became necessary to perform environmental surveys throughout the manufacturing facility. During these surveys thousands of samples were collected. All contamination found was subjected to Gram stains. Typical Gram-positive organisms were tracked and for some companies were identified. For all site, the Gram-negative organism were identified to genus and species. For some of the companies, only genomic identifications were performed for the Gram-negative isolates.

The data accrued in the environmental surveys was analyzed to determine where there were accumulations of Gram-negative organisms and specifically organisms that are part of the BCC group. Typically, these organisms were found in the water systems, standing water, and drain lines.

Once found, the next step was to remediate the contamination. Previous presentations indicated some resistance of these organisms to disinfectants and antibiotics (Ensor, 2017). Portable carts that generated ozonated water were utilized to decontaminate, disinfect, and in some instances, to sterilize the sources of contamination. Ozonated water is useful for the following reasons:

- Does not adversely affect the equipment surfaces, e.g., stainless steel.
- Can be validated for sterilization using USP < 1229 > with biological indicators.
- Can be qualified for disinfection efficacy to meet compendial requirements.
- Can be used at ambient conditions.
- Lower cost of use than many commercially available disinfectants.
- No indications of microorganism resistance to ozone.
- 12-logs of biological indicator can be eliminated in about 20 minutes.
- For sterile processes, depyrogenation can also be achieved at ambient conditions.

When used in drains, it also eliminates the odors emitted from the drain.

10.6.2.3   Results of Ozonated Water for Decontamination

All of the sites using ozonated water for decontamination were successful in eradicating the contamination present. Subsequent environmental surveys and product testing results showed that no BCC was present

10.7   CONCLUSION

It is important to be aware of potential sources for microbial contamination and conditions allowing for microbial proliferation. This can be accomplished by controlling raw materials, the manufacturing process and the manufacturing environment. It is useful to use quality-by-design techniques in designing and implementing the contamination control process (Ensor, 2017).

It may become necessary for more extensive microbial monitoring and identification of organisms to take place for non-sterile aqueous products, as a support system to ensuring that the product meets its final microbial release specifications.

LITERATURE CITED

Anderson, R. R., Warnick, P. and Scheckenberger, P. C. (1997) Recurrent CDC Group IVc-2 Bacteremia in a Human with AIDS. *Journal of Clinical Microbiology* (Mar) 35(3):780–782.

Aspinall, S., and Graham, R. (1989) Two Sources of Contamination of a Hydrotherapy Pool by Environmental Organisms. *Journal of Hospital Infection* 14:285–292.

Balada-Llasat, J-M, et al. (2010) Pseudo-Outbreak of *Cupriavidus pauculus* Infection at an Outpatient Clinic Related to Rinsing Culturette Swabs in Tap Water. *Journal of Clinical Microbiology* 48(7):2645–2647.

Brennan, Z. (2017) FDA to Drug Manufacturers: Beware Water-Borne Contaminants, RAPS. Downloaded from: http://raps.org/Regulatory-Focus/News/2017/05/22/27621/FDA-to-Drug-Manufacturers-Beware-Water-Borne-Contaminants/on January 2, 2018.

Clark, W. et al. (1984) Identification of Unusual Pathogenic Gram Negative Aerobic and Facultatively Anaerobic Bacteria. CDC, Atlanta, Georgia.

Code of Federal Regulations (CFR) (2017) The Code of Federal Regulations Title 21 – Food and Drugs. GMP Publications, Inc. The following chapters are noted throughout the document:

- 21 CFR 314.50(d)(1)
- 21 CFR 211.110
- 21 CFR 211.113(a)
- 21 CFR 211.160(b)
- 21 CFR 211.165
- 21 CFR 211.192
- 21 CFR 314.94(a)(9)

Coenye, T., Vandamme, P., and LiPuma, J. J. (2002) Infection by *Ralstonia* Species in Cystic Fibrosis Patients: Identification of *R. pickettii* and *R. mannitolilytica* by Polymerase Chain Reaction (Journal) *Emerging Infectious Diseases*; *Centers for Disease Control and Prevention* 8(7). Downloaded from wwwnc.cdc.gov/eid/article/8/7/01-0472_article.htm on July 15, 2013.

Ensor, L. A. (2017) Microbiological Quality Considerations in Non-sterile Pharmaceutical Product Manufacture. Presentation Given at the PDA European Pharmaceutical Microbiology Conference held in Porto, Portugal, on February 14–15, 2017.

Food and Drug Administration (FDA) (2017) FDA Advises Drug Manufacturers That Burkholderia Cepacia Complex Poses a Contamination Risk in Non-Sterile, Water-Based Drug Products. Downloaded from: www.fda.gov/Drugs/DrugSafety/ucm559 508.htm?source=govdelivery&utm_medium=email&utm_source=govdelivery   on January 2, 2017.

Kalka-Moli, W. M., et al. (2009) Airway Infection with a Novel *Cupriavidus* Species in Persons with Cystic Fibrosis. *Journal of Clinical Microbiology* (September) 47(9): 3026–3028.

LPSN (2013) List of Prokaryotic Names with Standing in Nomenclature. Downloaded from www.bacterio.cict.fr/c/cuprividus.html.

Manara, C. M. et al. (1990) Heterotrophic Plate Counts and the Isolation of Bacteria from Mineral Waters on Selective and Enrichment Media. *Journal of Applied Bacteriology* 69:871–876.

Mezher, M. (2016) Florida CMO Recalls All Lots of Liquid Drugs Due to Bacteria Outbreak. RAPS. Downloaded from: www.raps.org/Regulatory-Focus/News/2016/08/10/2556 3/Florida-CMO-Recalls-All-Lots-of-Liquid-Drugs-Due-to-Bacteria-Outbreak/on January 2, 2017.

MicrobeWiki (2013) Ralstonia paucula. Downloaded from http://microbewiki.kenyon.edu/ index.php/Ralstonia_paucula on July 15, 2013.

MicrobeWiki (2017) Burkholderia Cepacia Complex. Downloaded from: microbewiki.kenyon.edu on January 2, 2018.

Moissenet, D., et al. (2001) *Ralstonia paucula* (Formerly CDC Group IV c-2): Unsuccessful Strain Differentiation with PCR-Based Methods, Study of the 16 S–23 S Spacer of the rRNA Operon, and Comparison with Other *Ralstonia* Species (*R. eutropha*, *R. pickettii*, *R. gilardii*, and *R. solanacearum*). *Journal of Clinical Microbiology* (January) 39(1):381–384.

Moldenhauer, J., Ed. (2012) *Environmental Monitoring: A Comprehensive Manual* Volume 6. Chapter 12: The Problem of *Burkholderia cepacia*. PDA/DHI Publishers. Bethesda, MD.

Ori, S. et al. (1998) Microbial Contamination of Sterile Water in Japanese Hospitals. *Journal of Hospital Infection* 38:61–65.

Stovall, S. H. (2010) Nosocomial Transmission of *Cupriavidus pauculus* During Extracororeal Membrane Oxygenation. *ASAIO J.* (September/October) 56(5):486–487.

Tasbakan, M. S., et al. (2010) A Case of Ventilator-Associated Pneumonia Caused by *Cupriavidus pauculus. Microbiyol. Bul.* (January) 44(1):127–131.

Torbeck, L., et al. (2011) *Burkholderia cepacia:* This Decision is Overdue. *PDA Journal of Pharmaceutical Science and Technology* 65:535–543. Downloaded from www.fda.gov/downloads/AboutFDA/CentersOffices/CDER/UCM275569.pdf on May 2, 2017.

UniProt Consortium (2013) Species Cupriavidus pauculus. Downloaded from www.uniprot.org/taxonomy/82633 on July 15, 2013.

(USP) < 61>/<62 > Microbiological Examination of Non-sterile Products: Microbial Enumeration Tests and Tests for Specified Microorganisms.

(USP) Chapter < 1111 > Microbiological Examination of Non-Sterile Products: Acceptance Criteria for Pharmaceutical Preparations and Substances for Pharmaceutical Use)8 and Test Procedures.

Vandamme, P., et al. (1999) *Assignment of Centers for Disease Control group IVc-2 to the genus Ralstonia as Ralstonia paucula sp. nov. International Journal of Systematic and Evolutionary Microbiology* 49:663–669.

Vaneechoutte, M., et al. (2004). *Wautersia gen. nov.*, a Novel Genus Accommodating the Phylogenetic Lineage Including *Ralstonia eutropha* and Related Species, and Proposal of *Ralstonia [Pseudomonas] syzygii* (Roberts et al., 1990) comb. nov. *International Journal of Systematic and Evolutionary Microbiology* 54:317–327.

Wikipedia (2017) Burkholderia cepacia complex. Downloaded from: https://en.wikipedia.org/wiki/Burkholderia_cepacia_complex on January 2,2018,https://www.sciencedirect.com/science/article/pii/S1201971214016014

11 What Is Mold and Why Is It Important?

Brian G. Hubka and Jeanne Moldenhauer

CONTENTS

11.1 DEFINING MOLD

Questionnaires issued to students close to their high school graduation asked, "Whether fungi are plants?" or "Whether fungi are bacteria?" Fifteen students responded that fungi are plants. The remaining 150 students responded that fungi are bacteria. The teachers were astounded by how many thought that fungi are bacteria. Fungi are neither plants nor bacteria. They are eukaryotes and have the complex cell structures and abilities to make tissues and organs like higher organisms (Moore et al., 2011a).

Fungi, which include the organisms that are called yeasts and molds can have a very significant impact on human existence, e.g. (Moore et al., 2011a):

- The following would not be available without fungi: bread, alcohol, soft drinks, cheese, and coffee.
- Fungi can secrete enzymes into their environment to digest nutrients externally to start biotech processes such as cheese production.
- They aid in the digestion of grass eaten by cows.
- They make plant roots work more effectively helping to grow corn, oats, potatoes, lettuce, cabbage, peas, celery, herbs, spices, cotton, flax, timber, and the like.
- They aid in the production of oxygen for us to breathe.
- They produce a variety of compounds used to make medications such as cholesterol-controlling drugs (statins) and some antibiotics, e.g., penicillins and agricultural fungicides.
- They are even used in the distressing process of denim to manufacture stone-washed jeans.

Unfortunately, fungi are not always good for us. They can be responsible for diseases of crops, human infections, and can produce harmful chemicals like mycotoxins that can impact pharmaceuticals.

11.2   WHY ARE MOLDS IMPORTANT?

Product recalls due to mold have had high visibility in the industry. Several recalls of products due to mold contamination occurred, including the following (Cundell, 2016):

- Pharmaceutical tablet recalls in 2009 through 2011 due to the mold generated Tribromoanisole taints from wooden pallets. Lumber treated with Tribromophenol (TBP) in South America was used in the Caribbean. Due to the high humidity in Puerto Rico, mold growth occurred on the pallets. This in turn resulted in fungal methylation of TBP to the volatile, odorous taint tribromoanisole (TBA). Although users did not like the odor, it was not a toxicological concern. PDA Technical Report No. 55 (2017) was published regarding this topic.
- Sanofi Pasteur's 2012 Food and Drug Administration (FDA) Warning Letter for a sterile product manufacturing facility in Toronto, Canada due to mold contamination. This recall started with flooding that lead to water damage. Fungal colonies grew in the water damaged building materials. Although mold contamination was found, complete investigations and corrective actions were not adequately conducted.
- The New England Compounding Center (NECC) of Framingham, MA recalled three lots of steroid product (17,676 syringes) following a multistate outbreak of fungal meningitis caused by the mold *Exserohilium rostratum*.

In 2012, FDA inspected this compounding center and issued an FDA-483. The environmental monitoring data showed numerous environmental monitoring excursions out of limits. This facility was not operating in a state of control and resulted in 753 fungal meningitis infections, including over 60 deaths, across 20 states.

There are numerous health concerns with mold contamination in pharmaceutical manufacturing environments including: pathogenicity, allergic reactions, mycotoxins, and the invasiveness of mold (Hubka and Moldenhauer, 2015).

11.2.1 PATHOGENICITY

Some types of mold are inherently pathogenic. Natural Health Techniques (2015) has identified many types of fungi as pathogenic (Hubka and Moldenhauer, 2015). When performing risk assessments and product impact assessments relative to mold contamination one should include an assessment of the medical impact of this mold on patients and include the route of administration as a risk factor in the assessment.

11.2.2 MYCOTOXIN PRODUCTION

Mycotoxins are secondary toxic metabolites produced by fungi. These mycotoxins can be some of the most toxic substances in existence. There are at least 21 different mycotoxin classes with over 400 individual toxins produced by at least 350 fungi. Mycotoxins are potentially hazardous to man and animal health causing cancer and serious diseases. *Aspergillus, Fusarium, Penicillium*, and *Stachybotrys* are the major genera producing mycotoxins. There are several different types of mycotoxins. The types include (moldpedia.com, 2015; Hubka and Moldenhauer, 2015):

- Aflatoxins (AFT) are produced by *Aspergillus flavus* and *Aspergillus parasiticus* which are common contaminants in agricultural products. Based on their fluorescence under ultraviolet light (blue or green) and relative chromatogenic mobility during TLC analysis, B_1, B_2, G_1, and G_2 and M_1 and M_2 are the major AFT.
- Ochratoxin which includes Ochratoxin A, B, and C Ochratoxin A (OTA) is produced by some species such as *Aspergillus ochraceous* mainly in tropical regions and by *Penicillium verrucosum* in temperate ones.
- Trichothecene which is produced by *Stachybotrys* and includes Satratoxin-H, Vomitoxin, and T-2 mycotoxins
- Fumonisins include Fumonisin B1 and B2
- Zearalenone, an estrogenic mycotoxin produced by some Fusarium species causing problems in livestock production

It is very difficult to find a comprehensive identification of all the applicable mycotoxins. Table 11.1 identifies some of the mycotoxin producers. It is important to note that many different organisms have not been studied relative to the production of mycotoxins. As such, it is important to research individual isolates to determine if

TABLE 11.1

Toxin Producing Fungi

Fungal Identification	Mycotoxin(s) Produced
Acremonium species	Can product trichotecene, which is toxic if ingested.
Alternaria alternate	Capable of producing tenuazonic acid and other toxic metabolites.
Aspergillus candidus	It produces the toxin patulin and citrinin.
Aspergillus clavatus	It produces the toxin patulin.
Aspergillus flavus	Some species produce aflatoxins.
Aspergillus nidulans	It can produce the mycotoxin sterigmatocystin.
Aspergillus oschraceus	It can produce a kidney toxin that can result in oschratoxicosis in humans (aka "Balkan Nephropathy."
Aspergillus parasiticus	Strains of this species can produce mycotoxins in the aflatoxins group.
Aspergillus species	Many species may produce mycotoxins, dependent upon the food source and the fungus.
Aspergillus terreus	This species can produce the toxins patulin and citrinin.
Aspergillus versicolor	It can product mycotoxins, e.g., sterigmat ocystin and cyclopiaxionic acid.
Bipolaris species	This fungus can produce the mycotoxin – sterigmatocystin.
Chaetonium species	Can produce a mycotoxin called chaetoglobosin.
Eurotium species	The health effects and toxicity are closely related to that of the *Aspergillus* anamorph.
Fusarium solani	Can produce trichotecene toxins.
Fusarium species	Several species in this genus can produce potent trichlthecene toxins. Produces vomitoxin on grains.
Neosartorya species	The toxicity is closely related to the *Aspergillus* anamorphs.
Penicillium species	Some species can produce mycotoxins.
Scedosporium species	Two species of this organism cause health effects that can be fatal, *Scedosporium apiospermum* and *Scedosporium prolificans*. (The literature is not clear whether is this is a result of a toxin or not)
Stachybotrys species	Toxins produced include: macrocyclic trichotecenes, varracarin J, roridin E, Satratoxin F, G & H, Sporidesmin G, Trichoverrol, and Cyclosporins.

Source: Adapted from Moldenhauer, 2017a.

more updated data is available for that organism relative to the production of myco-toxins. It is also important to check more than one database, as different authors cite different sources of information.

Whether the mycotoxins are produced under the conditions in pharmaceutical manufacturing also will depend on the available substrates, pH and environmental conditions, these risk factors being particularly important in evaluation of molds found in the environment of pharmaceutical manufacturing.

Mycotoxins are not alive, so you can't "see them" on a culture plate. Eradicating mycotoxins involves the breaking down of the mycotoxin so that they are no longer dangerous to humans. Some of them are inactivated with 5% sodium hypochlorite, while others require high temperatures (260°C) for at least ten minutes for inactiva-tion. Ozone has been reported to inactivate most types of mycotoxins, however it requires a level of ozone that also has safety concerns for humans. HEPA air filters do not effectively remove mycotoxins (they are as small as 0.1 microns), although activated carbon filters are able to remove mycotoxins from the air. While mycotoxins can lose their toxicity over time, it may take several years to do this (moldpedia. com, 2015).

There is a scarcity of direct information of the potential presence of mycotoxins in medicines and their impact on patients. Such medicines would not be released to market since there is no routine release test for mycotoxins at this time. Reactions from food mycotoxins provide us with valuable information about the impact on animals and mycotoxins. There are even some test kits for various mycotoxins available for foods.

11.2.3 ALLERGIC REACTIONS

Some individuals have an overly sensitive immune system that responds to specific types of mold. When the mold spores are inhaled, the body recognizes them as foreign objects and develops allergy causing antibodies to be developed to fight off the foreign object. Following exposure, memory antibodies remain that can remember this foreign substance and respond to future attacks by this foreign substance. The immune system typically reacts to this response by release of substances like histamine. This in turn results in itchy, watery eyes, runny nose, sneezing, and other allergy symptoms (Mayo Clinic Staff, 2015; Hubka and Moldenhauer, 2015).

Some of the most common molds that generate allergic reactions include: *Alternaria, Aspergillus, Cladoporium*, and *Penicillium* (Mayo Clinic Staff, 2015).

A Mayo Clinic Study implicates fungus as cause of chronic sinusitis. In the Mayo Clinic Newsletter 1999, the researchers stated:

> An estimated 37 million people in the United States suffer from chronic sinusitis, an inflammation of the membranes of the nose and sinus cavity. Its incidence has been increasing steadily over the last decade. Common symptoms are runny nose, nasal congestion, loss of smell and headaches.

It also states: "Fungus allergy was thought to be involved in less than ten percent of cases," says Dr. Sherris. "Our studies indicate that, in fact, fungus is likely the cause of nearly all of these problems. And it is not an allergic reaction, but an immune reaction" (Hubka and Moldenhauer, 2015).

11.2.4 INVASIVENESS OF MOLD

The structure of molds and their spores allows for the spores to spread rapidly and linger in the environment. Since the spores are not defense mechanisms (like bacterial spores) but rather reproductive agents, the spores can provide for more growth of mold in a facility. In addition to growth due to spores, scientists have identified fungal propagules, which are structures that are used for the purpose of propagating an organism to the next stage in their life cycle (Hubka and Moldenhauer, 2015).

A hypha (plural hyphae) is a long, branching filamentous structure of a fungus. In most fungi, hyphae are the main mode of vegetative growth, and are collectively called a mycelium. Hyphae, which is the stick-like part that grows out of mold, are delicate and can break off even with a slight air current. These hyphal pieces are found to be very small and very viable and are referred to as propagules. Hyphal fragments or mycelia are components of fungal growth (like the roots and branches of a tree). It is common to find small hyphal fragments in outdoor air and in indoor dust. Propagules, which are units that can give rise to another organism, are important due to their small size, which can easily pass through a HEPA filter pore (Gorney, 2002; Hubka and Moldenhauer, 2015; Moldenhauer 2017c).

11.3   CRITERIA FOR MOLD GROWTH

Mold requires four things for growth: available mold spores (or propagules), food, the right temperature, and considerable moisture. Mold spores are ubiquitous – they are literally everywhere. Methods to reasonably and reliably eradicate them are not effective in the environment (not in a cleanroom). Attempting to eradicate mold by eliminating the presence of mold spores is deemed non-feasible (FSEC, 2015; Hubka and Moldenhauer, 2015).

Molds are not fussy eaters. If the other three requirements for growth are met, they can live on very few nutrients. Basically, they live off any carbon atoms (organic substances present). The oil remaining from your skin touching a surface can provide sufficient nutrients for the mold to grow if it is not properly removed during cleaning and disinfection. Even the soap used for cleaning can provide a nutrient for mold growth. Even items like wood, paper, and organic fibers can be used as nutrients (FSEC, 2015). Studies performed on the PVC material used to manufacture some IV bags showed that mold could obtain sufficient nutrients to grow from the IV bags alone as long as moisture is present. Because of the fungal ability to utilize so many nutrients it can be very difficult to control mold by eliminating their sources of nutrients (Hubka and Moldenhauer, 2015).

One thing many people overlook is that mold is fed by the microscopic pollen in the air. Pollen is a terrific mold nutrient, allowing mold to grow on glass with the right moisture present (Hubka and Moldenhauer, 2015).

Molds tend to grow at a variety of temperatures, from cold storage to those temperatures that are quite warm. It is common to find out that temperatures close to freezing (e.g., in a refrigerator) are not sufficiently cold to inhibit mold growth. Many believe that temperatures must be in the room temperature range (20° to 25°C) for mold growth. Molds grow quite well at 30° to 35°C also. They can cause disease in humans, which have normal body temperatures around 37°C. In fact, temperatures much warmer, like those in tropical regions are also conducive to mold growth (Hubka and Moldenhauer, 2015).

Most molds require moisture and it can be necessary in sufficient quantities for growth. Typically, mycologists refer to this moisture as water activity necessary for growth. The specific water activity level necessary is different for different species of mold. Most molds have levels that correspond to corresponding relative humidity of at least 70%. Most major mold outbreaks occur where porous, cellulose-type materials have been kept wet by liquid water or sustained condensation (FSEC, 2015). Water leaks provide major opportunities for mold growth to occur (Hubka and Moldenhauer, 2015). Table 11.2 (adapted from WHO, 2009) identifies the moisture levels required for growth of selected microorganisms in construction, finishing, and furnishing materials. In this document, the WHO organization has classified fungi based upon the water activity and relative humidity levels needed for the organisms to proliferate.

The mold categories are defined by WHO as (1) primary colonizers, which can grow at a water activity less than or equal to 0.80; (2) secondary colonizers, which grow at a water activity level of 0.80–0.90; and (3) tertiary colonizers, which require a water activity greater than 0.90 to germinate and start mycelial growth (WHO, 2009).

Below are some points to consider for mold investigations (examples of potential root causes):

- Evidence of decaying or dead plant-based materials and visible soil.
- Interior areas with high levels of humidity or moisture with niches for potential growth (examples: cellulose-based building materials, HVAC systems, humidifiers, unsealed containers, or wall panels).
- Spreading of spores by water droplets and/or airflow patterns.
- Materials transfer, disinfection procedures using chemical agents that are ineffective versus mold spores.
- Potential cracks, leaks, standing water.
- Damaged articles that cannot be thoroughly cleaned and dried.
- Damaged HEPA filters.
- Trending of one or two predominant mold ID's typically indicates mold growing within the building, rather than coming in from an outside source.
- Mechanical structural vibration (disturbances indoors or outdoors).
- Areas with potential for high humidity that remain covered or in the dark.

11.3.1 PRODUCT IMPACT ANALYSIS

Thorough and complete investigations should be conducted when mold counts are out-of-limits. Sometimes, we tend to downplay the effect of higher counts and just release the product. It is important to understand how your product is used, and the likelihood for pathogenicity, allergenicity, mycotoxin production, and the invasiveness of the product. All these considerations should be discussed in the impact assessment, prior to release of the affected batches.

11.4   MOLD DETECTION AND IDENTIFICATION

11.4.1   MOLD DETECTION

Mold is typically found in pharmaceutical processes as part of the environmental monitoring results, product bioburden testing results, and may be visible on surfaces, e.g., due to water leaks or incomplete housekeeping.

TABLE 11.2
Moisture Levels Required for Growth of Selected Microorganisms in Construction, Finishing, and Furnishing Materials

Moisture Level	Category of Microorganism
High ($a_w > 0.90$; ERH > 90%)	Tertiary Colonizers (Hydrophilic)
	• *Alternaria alternate*
	• *Aspergillus fumigatus*
	• *Epicoccum* spp.
	• *Fusarium moniliforme*
	• *Muco plumbeus*
	• *Phoma herbarum*
	• *Phialophora* spp.
	• *Rhizopus* spp.
	• *Stachybotrys chartarum* (*S. atra*)
	• *Trichoderma* spp.
	• *Ulocladium consortiale*
	• *Rhodotorula* spp.
	• *Sporobolomyces* spp.
	• Actinobacteria (or Actinomycetes)
Intermediate (a_w 0.80–0.90; ERH 80% – 90%)	Secondary Colonizers
	• *Apergillus flavus*
	• *Asperfillus versicolor*
	• *Cladosporium cladosporioides*
	• *Cladosporium herbarum*
	• *Cladosporium sphaerospermum*
	• *Mucor circinelloides*
	• *Rhizopus oryzae*
Low ($a_w < 0.80$; ERH < 80%)	Primary Colonizers (xerophilic)
	• *Alternaria citri*
	• *Aspergillus* (*Eurotium*) *amsterdami*
	• *Aspergillus candidus*
	• *Aspergillus* (*Eurotium*) *glaucus*
	• *Aspergillus niger* (*aka Aspergillus brasiliensis*)
	• *Apergillus penicilliodes*
	• *Aspergillus* (*Eurotium*) *repens*
	• *Aspergillus restrictus*
	• *Aspergillus versicolor*
	• *Paecilomyces variotii*
	• *Penicillium aurantiogriseum*
	• *Penicillium brevicompactum*
	• *Penicillium chrysogenum*
	• *Penicillium commune*
	• *Penicillium expansum*
	• *Penicillium griseofulvum*
	• *Wallernia sebi*

Source: Adapted from WHO, 2009.

Following the recalls due to fungal contamination mentioned earlier, many pharmaceutical industry professionals re-evaluated their positions regarding mitigation of fungal contamination risk and may have found the following (Cundell, 2016):

- Failure to provide sufficient attention to fungal isolation and trending during environmental monitoring.
- Lack of knowledge on whether disinfection efficacy studies adequately mitigated risk of fungal contamination (e.g., is it effective against fungal spores?).
- Not understanding the concerns associated with water leaks in the facility and their impact on fungal populations.
- Not having sufficient equipment and/or technique to identify fungal contaminants to genus and/or species.

11.4.2 SELECTIVE MEDIA

There are several selective media useful to recover fungal contaminants; see Table 11.3 (Cundell, 2016).

11.4.3 INCUBATION CONDITIONS

Incubation to recover mold isolates is a subject with many different opinions. For many years, pharmaceutical companies have utilized two different media for sampling the environment. One media was designated for the isolation of bacteria and another media was chosen to selectively isolate fungi (yeast and molds). These media were typically incubated at 30°–35°C for a specified number of days for bacteria and at 20°–25°C for a specified number of days for fungi. It is also acceptable to incubate one standard agar (e.g., soybean casein digest agar) at dual temperatures, to be able to adequately recover bacteria and yeast and mold in the manufacturing environment using the same agar plate and therefore the same location.

In 1998, Marshall et al. published an article "Comparative Mold and Yeast Recovery Analysis (The Effect of Differing Incubation Temperature Ranges and Growth Media)", which evaluated the use of a single type of media for the collection of both bacteria and fungi and specified a set of incubation parameters that included the use of two-temperature ranges.

USP < 1116>, Microbiological Evaluation of Clean Rooms and Other Controlled Environments (current version) was revised in 2012 and indicates that when using two-temperature incubation of environmental monitoring plates, one should first incubate at the higher temperature (e.g., 30°–35°C) to ensure recovery of Gram-positive cocci, followed by incubation at the lower temperature (e.g., 20°–25°C). This chapter was subsequently updated to only be applicable to aseptic facilities, but the concepts may still apply to other manufacturing areas.

The media used in typical environmental monitoring evaluations may or may not contain neutralizing agents, such as polysorbate 80 and/or lecithin, to improve the recovery of microorganisms from areas that may have been exposed to sanitizers and disinfectants.

TABLE 11.3
No caption

Fungal Media	Description	Where Used/Comments
Corn Meal Agar (CMA)	Media with high cellulose content.	Recommended for the isolation of *Stachybotys chartarum*.
Dichloran-Glycerol Agar 18 (DG18)	Medium containing 18% glycerol used for the recovery of xerophilic yeast and mold.	This media is used for xerophilic fungal isolation.
Malt Extract Agar (MEA)	Gold standard medium for isolation and speciation in mold-contaminated buildings.	This media is recommended for general fungal isolation for indoor air monitoring mold contaminated buildings. Studies conducted over five years, showed higher mold counts compared to monitoring with TSA alone, when monitoring the exact same sites. However, it is not clear if the shorter incubation time and different temperature were the real issue.
Potato Dextrose Agar (SDA)	General purpose medium for the isolation of mold.	General purpose media used for mold isolation.
Sabouraud Dextrose Agar (SDA)	Medium for the isolation of dermatophytes. Recommended for total combined yeast and mold counts in USP<61>.	Widely used in pharmaceutical companies for mold isolation.
Trypticase Soy Agar (TSA)	Routine media used by many pharmaceutical companies for environmental monitoring.	Controlled Environmental Testing Association (CETA) recommended use of this single medium for monitoring in compounding pharmacies.
V8 Agar/V9 Agar[a]	Developed in 1965 as part of a research project, V9 Agar was noted to induce early sporulation in environmentally isolated yeasts and molds when compared with peptone and sugar-based formulas. The primary ingredients of the media are V8™ Juice and potatoes, thus the name V9 Agar. The naturally low pH makes the media inhibitory to most bacteria. Some continue to call it V8 agar.	Recommended for *Stachybotrys* and *Chaetomium* species.

[a] Cundell (2016) identifies this media as V8, but other sources identify this media as V9.

Gebala and Sandle (2013) compared a variety of fungal recovery media and found the best recovery results using Sabouraud dextrose agar (SDA).

Gordon et al. (2014) compared the different incubation conditions used for environmental monitoring and found that they had better results using two separate media Trypticase Soy Agar (TSA) and SDA and two incubation conditions.

The use of two types of agar plates in an aseptic area may not be possible due to space available, so the single agar at dual incubation may be preferable.

Since there is no single consensus on this subject, it is useful and important for a company to have a validation protocol that shows the efficacy of their environmental monitoring recovery, incubation conditions and media used from data generated in actual in-use conditions, not laboratory studies. Guidance on these types of studies is provided in Moldenhauer (2014).

11.4.4 MOLD IDENTIFICATION

When mold is detected, it is important to determine the identity of the mold found. Many companies use traditional morphology and microscopic evaluation as the only method of identification. The correct identification is dependent upon not only how it looks but the age of the culture and the method of incubation. It was not possible to utilize some of the automated systems for identification. As such, this led to many conflicting results, and improper identifications. It is not appropriate to only use morphology for identification in pharmaceutical microbiology laboratories today.

If classical methods are used, it is important to utilize experienced mycological expertise (Cundell, 2016).

Today, many systems can detect mold automatically. Some of these methods utilize proteolytic or genotypic methods.

The classification systems utilized in the 1950s and 1960s, did not properly deal with fungi protists and bacteria. Whitaker (1969) published a new classification scheme with five kingdoms: Animalia, Plantae, Fungi, Protista (eukaryotic microorganisms and a mixed grouping of protozoa and algae), and Monera (prokaryotic microorganisms, bacteria, and archaea). This system was widely accepted in the 1970s. There is a fundamental difference in the four eukaryotic kingdoms and the prokaryotes. The higher organism traits of eukaryotes include nuclei, cytoskeletons, internal membranes, and mitotic/meiotic division cycles (Moore et al., 2011b).

A later breakthrough by Carl Woese (1987) identified that all organisms contain small subunit rRNA (SSU rRNA). They were given this name (SSU rRNA) because they form a small subunit of a ribosome. Woese further believed that the SSU rRNA would be a perfect candidate for the universal chronometer of all life (Moore et al., 2011b).

Woese studied the relationships between different SSU rRNA gene sequences from different organisms. This resulted in many questions about the common beliefs used in the relationships between organisms. Several considerations were made for the phylogenetic studies, e.g. Moore et al. (2011b):

- They must be universally distributed across the group chosen for study.
- They must be functionally homologous.

- They change in sequence at a rate proportionate with the evolutionary distance to be measured (the broader the phylogenetic distance being measured, the slower must be the rate at which the sequence changes).

Table 11.4 from Moore et al., (2011b) describes the ribosomal rRNA sequences used in the identification of fungi.

The study of cladistics is a method that aims to reconstruct the genealogical descent of organisms through objective and repeatable analysis leading to a natural classification or phylogeny. It results in the tree-branching diagram (called a cladogram or phylogenetic tree) that shows the pattern of relationships between the organisms based on the characters used (Moore et al., 2011b).

It is extremely useful to have personnel at your site that are familiar with reading phylogenetic trees, who can interpret if you have similar or totally different sources of contamination.

Matrix Assisted Laser Desorption Ionization-Time of Fight (Maldi-TOF) is a proteonomic method (aka proteolytic method) of fungal identification that is available. This method is useful as it is very accurate, inexpensive, and rapid. It is a type of mass spectroscopy. Some companies utilize this type of identification system alone to perform the necessary identification.

If desired, this proteomic method may also be subjected to a genotypic identification, especially if there is a product failure involved. rRNA sequencing methods have been found to be more timely and accurate in fungal identifications (Cundell, 2016).

The data obtained, including the identification should be maintained and trended to evaluate whether there are trends occurring in the facility.

TABLE 11.4

Ribosomal rRNA Sequences Used to Identify and Classify Fungi

rRNA molecule	Structural rRNA?	Transcribed?	Level of Conservation	Taxa That Can Be Distinguished
18 S r RNA (Small subunit RNA)	Yes	Yes	Highly conserved domains interspersed with conserved domains	From domains to classes
5 S rRNA	Yes	Yes	Conserved domains	Classes and orders
28 S r RNA (large subunit RNA)	Yes	Yes	Conserved domains interspersed with variable domains	From phyla to species
Internally transcribed spacers (ITS) 1 and 2	No	Yes	Variable domains	Species and closely-related genera
Intergenic spacer (IGS)	No	Yes	Highly variable domains	Strains and races

11.5 SETTING LIMITS FOR MOLD CONTAMINATION

Establishing the appropriate mold limits is based upon several different factors, one of which is the manufacturing process type (Moldenhauer, 2017b). There is an unfortunate trend among some companies to develop a zero-tolerance for mold contamination. This is not scientifically sound or appropriate in most cases (Akers and Lindsay, 2014).

11.5.1 ASEPTIC PROCESSES

The FDA's Aseptic Processing Guidance (2004), United States Pharmacopeia (USP) < 1116>, and Eudralex Volume 4 Annex 1 identify limits for classified manufacturing areas used for aseptic processing. The limits established for these areas are very low. Should mold be present as part of this count, it may be necessary to perform an investigation into the source and remediation. (Akers and Lindsay, 2014)

This is not to say that mold is desirable in these processes, it is not. Depending upon the source of the contamination, mold remediation may be difficult and expensive (Akers and Lindsay, 2014).

Any mold found in Grades A and B areas should be considered an excursion and investigated.

11.5.2 NON-STERILE PROCESSES

Fortunately, there is compendial guidance in Pharm Europa 5.1.4 and USP <1111> and <1115> of acceptable mold counts for product bioburden. These limits can be useful in establishing limits for environmental monitoring limits, which currently do not have compendial limits. It is important to note that neither compendia expect a zero-tolerance for mold contamination!

Pharm Europa includes tables 5.1.4.1 and 5.1.4.2 – Acceptance criteria for microbiological quality of non-sterile dosage forms. This table includes a column entitled TYMC, i.e., total yeast and mold count, (CFU/g or CFU/mL). In this column the allowable counts range for 10^1–10^4 depending upon the route of administration for the product. As such, in setting limits one must understand the route of administration for the affected products and set the limits based upon the tightest regulatory limits required. Within the text of the monograph, there is a definition of what the CFU limits are where (Pharm Europa, 2017):

- 10^1 CFU means a maximum acceptable count of 20.
- 10^2 CFU means a maximum acceptable count of 200.
- 10^3 CFU means a maximum acceptable count of 2000, and so forth.

The United States Pharmacopeia <1115> (USP, 2017) states:

"Bioburden levels in the ranges of those recommended in *Microbiological Examination of Nonsterile Products: Acceptance Criteria for Pharmaceutical Preparations and Substances for Pharmaceutical Use*, USP<1111> are recognized as safe and do not

pose risk of infection or microbial toxins. Manufacturers should have a clear understanding of situations that could favor microbial growth within their facilities and
materials and should implement practical countermeasures."

The USP <1115> has similar tables (see Tables 11.1 and 11.2) to the *Pharm
Europa*. The range of allowable mold counts is from 10^1 to 10^3 depending upon the
route of administration for the product. It also has a similar method of interpreting
the maximum acceptable count for each CFU (USP, 2017; Moldenhauer, 2017b).

When you have the acceptable limits that can be in your bioburden with information that that level of contamination is considered SAFE, you can conduct a risk assessment of how much impact the environment has on your product, e.g., is it a closed or
open system; the inherent mold count in the product; and your company's comfort level
of control to set a limit that is the same or lower than the compendial guidance. One
may find it difficult to support limits higher than those in the compendia without supporting design, environmental, and product data (Moldenhauer, 2017b).

11.5.3 WORLD HEALTH ORGANIZATION (WHO)

The World Health Organization (WHO) has issued numerous guidelines relative to
pharmaceutical products as well as to other aspects of life, including those on indoor
air quality (WHO, 2000 and 2009). For indoor air quality, the guidance indicates
many health risks associated with exposure to molds and provides clinical evidence
of health exposure to molds (see the referenced appendices for each document).
While not specifying limits to be met, there are applicable requirements and guidance to establishing limits.

The World Health Organization (WHO) has issued indoor air quality guidelines
including, "The right to healthy indoor air" and in Principle 6 it says, "Under the principle of accountability, all relevant organizations should establish explicit criteria for
evaluating and assessing building air quality and its impact on the health of the population and on the environment" (WHO, 2000). In this guidance, there are specific
instructions as to actions to follow to ensure appropriate air quality inside of a building.

11.6 MOLD REMEDIATION METHODS

In accordance with the WHO (2009) guidance on indoor air quality "the presence
of many biological agents in indoor environments is attributable to dampness and
inadequate ventilation." Dampness is specifically attributed as contributing to both
microbiological and chemical contamination in the area, which can result in health
risks. As discussed earlier in this chapter, different mold types require different levels of humidity and water activity for growth. Some contaminants are a result of
molds being brought into the area, called transient contaminants, and others are a
result of the conditions within the area (see Table 11.2 earlier) called inherent contaminants. In Table 11.2 provided earlier there are differences between the primary,
secondary, and tertiary colonizers. As such, you can look at the organism identification and determine for inherent contamination the water levels present. This can aid
in determining whether you have an "unknown" leak or other issue to be resolved.

Once mold is detected in the facility, the task of remediation begins. Many focus on the task thinking of mold spores as being the same as bacterial spores. Bacterial spores are single walled cells, usually formed in response to hardship of some kind, and allow for survival of the cell after the hardship is resolved. Mold spores are tiny reproductive structures. They are made to germinate and multiply.

Not all mold is equal and therefore remediation methods may be different based upon the mold identification. One of the main considerations is looking for the source and eliminating it, because disinfection will only remove what is present, not what continues to be generated from the source. There are many publications by Jim Polarine and Paul Lopilito on fungal contaminations that are easier and/or more difficult to remediate (Barnett et al., 2007).

As such, it is useful to have disinfectant efficacy studies that show the effectiveness of your cleaning agents against the types of molds routinely recovered in your facility. Understanding the ability of the disinfectant to work for you is key, when routinely using disinfectants to remediate mold. It is also important to perform ongoing analysis of the surface environmental monitoring data to evaluate if new or recurring molds are found.

When you have visible mold on a wall or equipment surface, the concentration of mold present is likely very high. As such, the typical two or three-log reduction seen in a disinfection study may not be sufficient to eradicate the amount of mold present.

Some consultants indicate the need for 3X or 9X cleaning regimens to remediate a contaminated environment. These may or may not be effective, depending upon the disinfectants used, how they are used, the level of contamination present and so forth. The best remediation is prevention of mold contamination before it occurs! Or discovery of the source and eliminating it!

11.6.1 CONTAMINATED BUILDING FACILITIES

When you have problems in cleanrooms or testing areas due to seasonal or environmental molds, solutions like the use of ozone gas, chlorine dioxide gas, or nitrogen dioxide gas may be useful in decontaminating the facility. These methods can be effective in killing the mold and mold spores present, however if you continue to expose the environment to contaminated environmental air the area will quickly re-contaminate. As such, it may be necessary to routinely use this type of decontaminant until the "seasonal" contamination issue has passed. Some companies routinely implement these programs at a specified frequency in specified seasons. For example, a company may utilize monthly decontamination cycles from spring until fall. Caution should be taken when using fumigants too frequently, as they do generate moisture and may actually add to suitable conditions for growth, if the source of the mold has not been eliminated.

Water damage due to leaks or other sources should be immediately addressed. Part of the corrective action should include an assessment of the risk of mold contamination and preventative measures should be utilized to reduce this risk. High levels of mold in the facility and/or presence of specific harmful molds may require use of a certified technician to remove the mold and certify that the facility is safe for use by humans.

11.6.2 CONTAMINATED EQUIPMENT AND/OR SURFACES

Like facilities, one can choose to utilize a cleaning and disinfection method to reduce contamination. Since many cleaning and disinfecting agents can have an adverse effect on the equipment surfaces, it may be useful to consider newer non-traditional methods, e.g., the use of ozonated water to decontaminate.

The gaseous options provided for building decontamination (e.g., chlorine dioxide or ozone) can also be useful for transient mold contaminants. It is only effective for inherent contamination, if the gas can penetrate the area where the mold is present. Note: It is also important to fix the conditions that allowed for inherent mold to be present.

11.6.3 CONTAMINATED PRODUCT

In most cases, remediation of the product may not be possible unless your regulatory submission provides for some type of product reprocessing, or downstream steps can demonstrate removal of the mold and any potential mycotoxins. Key considerations in responding to the contamination include: a root cause analysis of where the contamination came from, corrective actions to eliminate the source of contamination, and preventative actions to prevent recurrence.

After that, the issues arise in determining whether the product is safe for use or should be rejected. A product impact analysis should be conducted, keeping in mind the various health risks associated with mold as well as GMP and quality requirements.

11.7 MOLD PREVENTION METHODS

The best way to deal with mold is to ensure it is NOT a contaminant in your process! It is like that adage, "an ounce of prevention is worth a pound of cure."

There are several different technologies available to prevent the likelihood of contamination starting with facility design. Appropriate engineering controls should be used in the design to prevent leaking, water or condensation build up, and the like. Where there is the potential for standing water or wetness, there is the potential for mold.

When doing reconstruction or repair procedures, it is important to realize that outside air has the potential for area contamination and mold spores. As such, appropriate safeguards should be put into place to prevent this air from contacting production areas. It is also important to respond quickly to the need for repairs for water damage in the facility.

A good defense for building materials is to use antimicrobial products for mold prevention during the construction process. Facilities that utilize antimicrobial flooring product protection, antimicrobial paint product technology, and stain-resistant bathroom fixtures can help prevent the growth of mold and mildew. These types of concerns can be important as building materials often contain starches, organic adhesives, and cellulose sugars, which are an ideal nutrient sources for mold (Microban, 2017).

An example of the antimicrobial product is manufactured by Microban®. Some of the products for prevention include: mold inhibiting window coverings, odor-resistant air filtration systems, antimicrobial flooring, sink and sealant products, and the like (Microban, 2017).

There are antimicrobial (and antifungal) paints available that can be used in locker rooms, change rooms, and other painted areas in the facility. Many of these products are based upon the use of silver nanoparticles. The types of areas where counts are typically high may have no counts or deeply reduced counts following application of the antimicrobial paints.

CASE STUDY ON MOLD (FALCO 2017):

- Environmental Monitoring Event: Atypical levels of mold were recovered from environmental monitoring test samples in a Grade D environment.
- Root Cause: Adjacent room outside the classified area in an access room to the decontamination autoclave had recovery of same mold in cracks in walls.
- Corrective Actions: Cracks in the walls in the access room where mold was found were sealed and repaired, then cleaned, and disinfected. A mold prevention solution (e.g., MoldGuardian™) was applied to the adjacent, non-classified area walls and floors.
- Effectiveness check on corrective actions and preventative measures: Atypical levels of mold have not been recovered in the manufacturing facility post changes.

11.8 CONCLUSION

There is a heightened awareness of molds in the pharmaceutical manufacturing environment and process due to some very high consequence cases in the past few years, including the NECC case that resulted in over 60 deaths and over 700 fungal infections from a contaminated injectable product. Environmental monitoring methods must be able to recovery molds routinely. Molds themselves not only can contaminate products, but they also may produce a variety of mycotoxins that cannot be detected by traditional release testing requirements, so products are rejected when mold is present. The presence of molds may indicate conditions within the manufacturing environment that can be a potential source that must be eliminated or may be coming from outside such as construction or inadequate air handling. There are a variety of methods that can be used to detect molds, either visually and manually, or by use of proteolytic or genotypic methods. Remediation of areas where molds have been found can include use of disinfectants, repairs of leaks, replacement of wet building materials, segregation of construction areas, and chemical guards to prevent molds from colonizing on surfaces.

LITERATURE CITED

Akers, J. and Lindsay, J. (2014) Determining Mold Facility Infection. *Pharmaceutical Technology* 38(10). Digital Edition. Downloaded from: www.pharmtech.com/determining-facility-mold-infection on May 8, 2017.

Barnett, C., Polarine, J., and Lopolito, P. (2007) Control Strategies for Fungal Contamination in Cleanrooms. *Controlled Environments* Magazine On-Line. Downloaded from: www.cemag.us/article/2007/09/control-strategies-fungal-contamination-cleanrooms on October 10, 2017.

Cundell, T. (2016) Mold Monitoring and Control in Pharmaceutical Manufacturing Areas. *American Pharmaceutical Review.* Downloaded from: www.americanpharmaceutica lreview.com/Featured-Articles/190686-Mold-Monitoring-and-Control-in-Pharmac eutical-Manufacturing-Areas/on May 30, 2017. 21 pages.

Falco, L. (2017) Case Study of Environmental Mold Isolation in a Controlled Manufacturing Facility, PDA 12th Annual Microbiology Conference.

Florida Solar Energy Center (FSEC) (2015) Mold Growth. Downloaded from: www.fsec.u cf.edu/en/consumer/buildings/basics/moldgrowth.htm on January 29, 2015.

Gebala, B. and Sandle, T. (2013) Comparison of Different Fungal Agar for the Environmental Monitoring of Pharmaceutical-Grade Cleanrooms. *PDA Journal of Pharmaceuticals Science and Technology* 67(6): 621–633.

Gordon, O., Berchtold, M., Staerk, A., and Roesti, D. (2014) Comparison of different incubation conditions for microbiological environmental monitoring. *PDA Journal Pharmaceutical Science and Technology* 68(5): 384–406.

Gorney, R. (2002) Fungal Fragments as Indoor Air Biocontaminants. *Applied Environmental Microbiology* 68(7): 3522–3531.

Hameed, A. A., Ayesh, A.M., Mohamed, A.R., and Mawalay, H.F.A. (2012) Fungi and Some Mycotoxins Producing Species in the Air of Soybean and Cotton Mills: A Case Study. *Atmospheric Pollution Research* 3(1): 125–131.

Hubka, B. G. and Moldenhauer, J. (2015) *Microbial Risk and Investigations.* PDA/DHI Publishers. Bethesda, MD.

Kielpinski, G., Prinzi, S., Duguid, J., and du Moulin, G. (2005) Roadmap to Approval: Use of an Automated Sterility Test Method as a Lot Release Test for Carticel, Autologous Cultured Chondrocytes. *Cytotherapy* 7(6): 531–541.

Marshall, V., Poulson-Cook, S., and Moldenhauer, J. (1998) Comparative Mold and Yeast Recovery Analysis (The Effect of Differing Incubation Temperature Ranges and Growth Media). *PDA Journal of Science and Technology* 52(4): 165–169.

Mayo Clinic Staff (2015) Diseases and Conditions: Mold Allergy: Causes. Downloaded from: http://www.mayoclinic.org/diseases-conditions/mold-allergy/basics/causes/con-200 25806 on January 29, 2015.

Microban (2017) Building Materials: Antimicrobial Products for Mold Prevention. Downloaded from: www.microban.com/micro-prevention/applications/building-mate rials on June 1, 2017.

Moldenhauer, J. (2014) Justification for Incubation Conditions Used for Environmental Monitoring. Downloaded from: http://www.americanpharmaceuticalreview.com/F eatured-Articles/158825-Justification-of-Incubation-Conditions-Used-for-Environm ental-Monitoring/on May 31, 2017.

Moldenhauer, J. (2017a) Personal Laboratory Information (not published).

Moldenhauer, J. (2017b) Setting Limits for Mold Contamination. *GXP Journal On Line.* 21(4). Downloaded from: http://www.ivtnetwork.com/gxp-journal on July 26, 2017.

Moldenhauer, J. (2017c) *Fungal Dictionary.* Contamination Prevention Technologies, Inc., Las Vegas, NV.

moldpedia.com (2015) Mycotoxins. Downloaded from: https://moldpedia.com/mycotoxins on January 29, 2015.

Moore, D., Robson, G. D., and Trinci, P. J. A. (2011a) *21st Century Guidebook to Fungi.* Cambridge University Press, Cambridge, UK, 1–17.

Moore, D., Robson, G. D., and Trinci, P. J. A. (2011b) *21st Century Guidebook to Fungi.* Cambridge University Press, Cambridge, UK, 18–40.

Natural Health Techniques (2015) List of Pathogenic Fungus, Molds, Mildews. Downloaded from: http://naturalhealthtechniques.com/list-of-pathogenic-fungi-molds-and-milde ws.htm on January 29, 2015.

Whitaker, R. H. (1969) New Concepts of Kingdoms of Organisms. *Science* 163: 130–161.

Woese, C. R. (1987) Bacterial Evolution. *Microbiological Reviews* 51: 221–271.

World Health Organization (WHO) (2000) *The Right to Healthy Indoor Air: Report on a Working Group Meeting, Bilthoven, The Netherlands, 15–17 May 2000.* Copenhagen, WHO Regional Office for Europe. Downloaded from: www.euro.who.int/document/ e69828.pdf on March 15, 2009.

World Health Organization (WHO) (2009) WHO Guidelines for Indoor Air Quality: Dampness and Moulds. WHO Regional Office – Europe. Downloaded from: www.e uro.who.int/__data/assets/pdf_file/0017/43325/E92645.pdf?ua=1 on October 10, 2017.

12 Sterilization Methods

Jeanne Moldenhauer

CONTENTS

12.1 MICROBIOLOGICAL CONTROL STRATEGIES IN THE MANUFACTURE OF REGULATED PRODUCTS

A key consideration in the manufacture of regulated products is the determination of the desired quality attributes for the product and providing manufacturing processes that can produce these products with the desired quality attributes. Among the critical quality attributes are quality, identity, strength, purity, and safety. Microbiology is a key component in many of these attributes. For sterile products, the absence of microorganisms is essential. However, it is important to note that contamination control includes other microbial hazards like: microbial toxins, prions, viruses, bacteria, and fungi (Miller et al., 2008; Moldenhauer, 2014).

Since microorganisms are present in the air, on surfaces, in components, in raw materials, and on people, one must ensure that the contamination control program is established and used in a way to ensure that these organisms do not affect the final product quality. The company should conduct a formal evaluation of the potential sources of contamination, when and how they may occur, and the effect on product quality if contamination does occur. This evaluation typically starts in the product development phase and continues throughout the evaluation of the manufacturing process. Hazard analysis and critical control point (HACCP) (Food and Drugs Administration [FDA], 1997) and failure mode and effect analysis (FMEA) (Stamatis, 2003) methods can be useful in conducting this evaluation (Miller et al., 2008; Moldenhauer, 2014).

In a typical manufacturing process, the equipment used can contribute to the bioburden present in the product. Typical equipment can include: tanks, carboys, transfer lines, pumps, scrapers, mixers, and so forth (Miller et al., 2008). Depending upon the stage of production where the equipment is used, it is typically cleaned and sanitized and disinfected or sterilized prior to use. Some pieces of equipment are sterilized in bags or wraps that can maintain a microbial barrier following sterilization. Other items are too large or too heavy to move into a sterilizer and may be cleaned and sterilized in place, using a moist heat (steam) process. When the items are sterilized in place, part of the validation should include an evaluation of how long the item may be held post treatment and maintain its sterilized state (Moldenhauer, 2014).

People are frequently attributed to be the biggest source of microbial contamination in a pharmaceutical environment. Obviously, we can't sterilize the people to eliminate the contamination they carry. Instead we enclose them in sterile gown, gloves, boots, hair coverings, and masks to prevent the microorganisms they carry from entering the manufacturing environment. Purchased disposable gowning items like gloves are typically ethylene oxide or radiation sterilized. Other gases may also be used for sterilization. Most often reusable gowning items are moist heat (steam) sterilized. Wearing this gowning and use of meticulous aseptic technique is designed to prevent contamination of the product (Moldenhauer, 2014).

Manufacturing supplies (e.g., components, vials, seals) are at least cleaned and sanitized prior to use in the manufacturing area. Depending upon the type of product sterilization (e.g., aseptic versus moist or dry heat sterilization) these supplies may be sterilized before or after assembly (Moldenhauer, 2014).

Water used in the manufacturing process is typically not sterilized, however many companies maintain the water in a tank or loop at an elevated temperature to significantly reduce the bioburden present (Moldenhauer, 2014).

The actual manufacturing environment, e.g., the air in the area, is typically subjected to a rigorous, validated cleaning and sanitization process. Following this process, some companies choose to use products like vaporized hydrogen peroxide or peracetic acid to sterilize the area. Other companies choose to use monitoring to control the level of contamination present in the area. Today several systems are available that provide real time, or near real time monitoring results for viable biological particles in the air (Moldenhauer, 2014).

12.2 DEFINING STERILIZATION

Sterilization processes are used to destroy or eliminate the microorganisms that are present on the surfaces or materials to aid in providing a safe pharmaceutical product for the patient. All sterilization processes are intended to result in materials or surfaces that have become sterile, or free from viable microorganisms. While this dictionary definition of sterility sounds good, in the real world we do not have a way to routinely test or evaluate for the absence of all viable microorganisms in all samples (Agalloco, 2008; Moldenhauer, 2014).

When products are labeled sterile, the common assumption is that the vendor is claiming to meet the dictionary definition of sterility. This is further complicated by the fact that most sterile products are released using a national standard – the compendial sterility test methodology. It is common to assume that passing this test indicates that there are no viable organisms present. However, in 1956 Bryce identified two critical limitations of the compendial sterility test method. His first concern was that the viable organisms present in the test sample can only be cultivated if they are able to do so under the specific test conditions. Secondly, the number of samples tested is so small (it is a destructive test) that at best it can only be used to provide a gross estimate of the "sterility" of the test sample (Bryce, 1956; Moldenhauer, 2014).

Knudsen (1949) added to Bryce's comments, to indicate that the sample size is not of a statistically significant population to accurately estimate sterility. As such, the compendial sterility test is a poor indicator of test sample sterility. The ability to accurately detect contamination with a 95% confidence level is about 15% when using this test method. The probability of microorganisms surviving is 10^{-1} or 10%. While it is possible to improve these numbers by increasing the sample size, most have not considered this type of increase, because the test cost would increase. Since this is a destructive test, the test samples used in a statistically valid sample plan would be costly and possibly wasteful (DeSantis, 2008; Moldenhauer, 2014).

The sterility test method would be more reliable if one were able to detect single microorganisms, in-line, and without destroying the sample. At such a time when a method like this is available for commercial use the validity of the test may be greatly improved (Sutton and Moldenhauer, 2004; Moldenhauer, 2014).

Sterilization processes are utilized to eliminate the microbial contamination that may be present. Scientists have carefully researched the destruction of microorganisms (Agalloco, 2008). Defining when a cell is dead is a complex issue. In fact, no single definition exists of when a cell is dead. Many use the definition that the cell is unable to continue to replicate, but microbial cells can have long dormant phases. Some cells can form spores which are resistant to adverse conditions and exist in the spore state for very long periods of time. Some have even reported spores that have existed for hundreds of years. But, when the cell is exposed to favorable growth conditions these spores can be revived and replicate (Setlow, 2009). Some other microorganisms that are not able to form spores can form viable-but-non-culturable (VBNC) cells. Oliver et al. (1995) states many of the estimates of the number of microorganisms present in the environment are much lower than the real number of cells present. One of the problems in estimating counts is the capability to recover microorganisms is dependent upon the culture methods used.

Use of a sterilization process is to eliminate the viable microorganisms present, to a specified level of sterility assurance (SAL), which is also called the probability of a non-sterile unit (PNSU). Studies are performed to show that the sterilization process is effective. Generating the documentation to show effectiveness and control of the process is called validation. Good science and engineering practices are used to assess the functions and capabilities of the sterilization process (Moldenhauer, 2014).

Regulatory guidance is available from different agencies which indicate that manufacturers of pharmaceutical products are responsible for performing validation studies to ensure that the critical aspects of the system or operation are controlled and operating to perform their specified functions (European Union, 2001; FDA, 2003; Moldenhauer, 2014).

The definition of validation may not be identical in all documents, but all of them include requirements to provide documented evidence of the system's performance within specified parameters. Agalloco (1993) provides a definition that is comprehensive and descriptive: "Validation is a defined program which in combination with routine production methods and quality control techniques provides documented assurance that a system is performing as intended and/or that a product conforms to its predetermined specifications. When practiced in a 'life cycle' model it incorporates design, development, evaluation, operational and maintenance considerations to provide both operational benefits and regulatory compliance" (see also Moldenhauer, 2014).

12.3   WHAT IS THE DIFFERENCE BETWEEN STERILIZATION AND SANITIZATION?

Sanitization is defined as the destruction of microorganisms that may or may not be pathogenic, on surfaces using chemicals or heat. Sanitizing destroys the microorganisms however it may or may not achieve the same lethality offered by sterilization cycles. When using either of these terms, it is useful to clearly define the intended meaning within your documentation system (Moldenhauer, 2013 and 2014).

Some companies use the term sanitization when describing processes used to reduce bioburden, without needing all of the validation and documentation associated with a sterilization cycle. For example, the microorganisms may be destroyed, but the cycle is not designed nor expected to meet the same levels of sterility assurance as a validated sterilization cycle (Moldenhauer, 2013 and 2014).

12.4 KEY CONCEPTS FOR THE VALIDATION OF STERILIZATION PROCESSES

There are a variety of fundamental concepts of validation that are applicable when validating sterilization processes in pharmaceutical applications. Validation protocols should be based upon good science and engineering practices. The scientific method is used in designing and executing validation studies, typically documented in a protocol or series of protocols. This involves assessment of the critical performance aspects for the sterilizer and development of methods to evaluate this performance. The experiments are designed based upon the hypothesis developed (e.g., sterilization will be accomplished to a specific sterility assurance level). The testing is conducted to assess whether the hypothesis developed is or is not true. The observations made, and the results obtained lead to the development of a conclusion. The conclusion identifies whether the testing is acceptable (Agalloco, 2008; Moldenhauer, 2013 and 2014).

There is the expectation that testing will be conducted to verify that all critical parameters are met. This is accomplished using test equipment which is properly calibrated or qualified as appropriate. For calibrated equipment, the accuracy should be traceable to established national or international standards (Agalloco, 2008; Moldenhauer, 2013 and 2014).

Another expectation is for the reproducibility of the system's performance (consistency of performance). In the case of sterilization systems, it is expected that the performance be evaluated within a specific sterilization cycle as well as across a series of cycles (Agalloco, 2008). For sterilization, this includes a minimum of three consecutive acceptable cycles as part of the initial validation. An assessment should be conducted to determine the number of studies that should be performed to ensure appropriate testing has been conducted to demonstrate consistent and reliable performance of the system. For example, if you are qualifying both minimum and maximum load configurations it may be necessary to perform three studies each iguration (Moldenhauer, 2013 and 2014).

Worst case conditions are evaluated during the validation studies. Among the worst case conditions for sterilization, it is common to test at or below the minimum allowable conditions for exposure time and/or temperature. There is a trend in some companies to just run the validation studies at the nominal production cycles, however, in the event of a cycle that is at the lower acceptable specification limit, you may have no data to support the efficacy of the cycle (Moldenhauer, 2013 and 2014).

There is a concept that has developed over the years for sterilization: "the bugs don't lie." While this statement has been attributed to several different individuals, it is widely accepted in the pharmaceutical industry. This statement indicates that the microorganisms used as part of the test system evaluate the performance of the sterilizer process. Whether they live, or die is a reflection of all the conditions to which there were exposed during the sterilization cycle. For example, it possible to obtain thermal data that indicates an acceptable cycle was delivered to a sterilizer load, and yet they have biological indicator results which show that an unacceptable condition occurred. Over the years many have thought "there is something wrong with the biological indicators," when in reality the expected sterilization process was not delivered to all of the areas where the biological indicators were placed within the load (Moldenhauer, 2013 and 2014).

Similarly, another thought is generally accepted as true: "if it isn't documented, it didn't happen." It isn't enough to execute the validation studies; there must be documented evidence that the studies were conducted. The data should be accurate, legible, and generated in accordance with good manufacturing practices (GMPs) and the data must be maintained in a way that allows it to be found and reviewed whenever necessary. Keep in mind that this includes data from data acquisition studies. Older data acquisition equipment used 8" disks, 3.5" disks, various Windows Operating Systems, and so forth. Ensuring that these data are copied accurately and retrievability for many years requires the use of an established program to guarantee that these tasks are performed. Most sterilizer validation studies are documented as part of protocols or standard operating procedures (SOPs) (Moldenhauer, 2013 and 2014).

Validation of the sterilizer once is not enough. It must also be maintained in a validated state, including maintenance of the equipment, software, support systems, and such so that the validation state is maintained. There should be controls established to maintain the system in a state of control. Procedures should be established to monitor and evaluate changes made to the system, i.e. it should be part of a change control system. When changes are made, they should be reviewed to assess the impact on the validated state of the system. Preventative maintenance should be conducted to ensure that the system is maintained in "good" operating condition. Access to the system should be limited to appropriately qualified and trained individuals. It is typically not sufficient to only validate the system when changes are made. For most regulated industries there is an expectation that periodic validation or qualification of the sterilization system is also conducted (Moldenhauer, 2013 and 2014).

12.5 WHAT REGULATORY REQUIREMENTS MUST BE MET FOR STERILIZATION VALIDATION?

Since sterilization is a critical operation there are many regulatory expectations for the validation of these processes. Within these regulatory expectations there are differences in how the validation should be conducted and what parameters are most important in the validation (HTM-2010, 1994; FDA, 1984; EN285, 1997). It is important to understand the regulatory requirements for sterilization that must be met for your affected product and the countries in which the product is sold (Moldenhauer, 2013 and 2014).

In 1976, the FDA published the *Proposed Current Good Manufacturing Practices for Large Volume Parent,* which is also called the GMPs for large-volume parenterals (LVPs) (FDA, 1976). This document was drafted by the Agency in response to problems with sterility in LVPs, that resulted in the death or affected patients. While this document was withdrawn by FDA and never officially issued, many of the requirements within this document have become the small "c" ("current") in cGMPs relative to sterilization validation used for terminal sterilization. Some examples include: requirements for temperature distribution evaluations and heat penetration evaluations, calibration of instruments, use of biological indicators as part of the validation process, and worst-case evaluations (Agalloco, 2008; Moldenhauer, 2013 and 2014).

FDA has provided guidance for some types of sterilization processes, e.g., FDA's *Guidance for Industry Sterile Drug Products Produced by Aseptic Processing – cGMP* (2004). There are also numerous inspector guidance documents for how to look at and assess the sterilization processes used at various companies. In addition, there is a *Guidance for Industry for the Submission Documentation for Sterilization Process Validation in Applications for Human and Veterinary Drug Products* (FDA, 1994b).

The European Union has Annex 1 which includes information on this topic (EU GMPs, 2008). Additionally, there is a *Decision Trees for the Selection of Sterilisation Methods* (CPMP/QWP/054/98) (EMEA, 2000) There is a British Standard for Sterilization – Steam Sterilizers – Large Sterilizers, BS EN 285:2006+A2:2009 (EN, 2009). [Note: There is a corresponding document, EN 284 for small steam sterilizers.]

Additionally, organizations like the Parenteral Drug Association (PDA) have issued technical reports that reflect industry standards for validation. Among the PDA documents governing sterilization are (Moldenhauer, 2014):

- PDA Technical Report 1, Revised 2007, (TR 1) Validation of Moist Heat Sterilization Processes Cycle Design, Development, Qualification and Ongoing Control (2007).
- PDA Technical Report 3 (TR3) Validation of Dry Heat Sterilization and Depyrogenation Cycles (2013).
- PDA Technical Report 3 (Revised 2013b) Validation of Dry Heat Processes Used for Sterilization and Depyrogenation (2013b).
- PDA Technical Report 7 (TR7) Depyrogenation (1981).
- PDA Technical Report 48 (TR48) Moist Heat Sterilizer Systems: Design, Commissioning, Operation, Qualification, and Maintenance (2010).
- PDA Technical Report No. 61 Steam in Place (2013a).

The International Organization for Standardization (ISO) also has published a variety of documents for sterilization processes. In addition to sterilization, they have documents for calibration and biological indicators. Some of the ISO documents include (Moldenhauer, 2014):

- ISO 13408-2006(r)2012 Aseptic Processing of Health Care Products – Part 5: Sterilization in Place
- ISO 14160: 2011 Sterilization of Health Care Products – Liquid Chemical Sterilizing Agents for Single Use Medical Devices Utilizing Animal Tissues and Their Derivatives – Requirements for Characterization, Development, Validation and Routine Control of Sterilization Processes for Medical Devices
- ISO 17665-1:2006 Sterilization of Health Care Products – Moist Heat – Part 1. Requirements for the Development, Validation and Routine Control of a Sterilization Process for Medical Devices.

- ISO 17665-3:2013 Sterilization of Health Care Products – Moist Heat – Part 3: Guidance on the Designation of a Medical Device to a Product Family and Processing Category for Steam Sterilization
- ISO 20857:2010 Sterilization of Health Care Products – Dry Heat – Requirements for the Development, Validation and Routine Control of a Sterilization Process for Medical Devices
- ISO 25424:2009 Sterilization of Medical Devices – Low Temperature Steam and Formaldehyde –Requirements for Development, Validation and Routine Control of a Sterilization Process for Medical Devices
- ISO 11137 Sterilization of Health Care Products Package

The American National Standards organization has also identified some sterilization documents (Moldenhauer, 2014):

- ANSI/AAMI/ISO 13408-5:2006/(R)2012 Aseptic Processing of Health Care Products – Part 5: Sterilization in Place
- ANSI/AAMI/ISO TIR 17665-2: 2009 Sterilization of Health Care Products – Moist Heat – Part 2: Guidance on the Application of ANSI/AAMI/ISO 17665-1

The USP has also generated several documents on sterilization (some are issued and some are drafts at this time) (Moldenhauer, 2014):

- <1211 > Sterilization and Sterility Assurance of Compendial Articles (USP, 2013a)
- <1229 > Sterilization of Compendial Articles (USP, 2013a)
- <1229.1 > Steam Sterilization by Direct Contact (USP, 2017)
- <1229.2 > Moist Heat Sterilization of Aqueous Liquids (USP, 2013b)
- <1229.3 > Monitoring of Bioburden (USP, 2017)
- <1229.4 > Sterilizing Filtration of Liquids (USP, 2013a)
- <1229.5 > Biological Indicators for Sterilization (USP, 2017)
- <1229.6 > Liquid Phase Sterilization (USP, 2013b)
- <1229.7 > Gaseous Sterilization (USP, 2013c)
- <1229.8 > Dry Heat Sterilization (USP, 2013d)
- <1229.9 > Physicochemical Integrators and Indicators for Sterilization (USP, 2017)
- <1229.10 > Radiation Sterilization (USP, 2013e)
- <1229.11 > Vapor Phase Sterilization (USP, 2017)
- <1229.12 > New Sterilization Methods (USP, 2017)
- <1229.13 > Sterilization in Place (USP, 2017)
- <1229.14 > Sterilization Cycle Development (USP, 2017)
- <1229.15 > Sterilizing Filtration of Gases (USP, 2017)

All the documents from regulatory agencies and industry are living documents. They change over time to reflect current expectations for sterilization validation. Some of these documents have conflicting requirements or different requirements than other documents (Moldenhauer, 2014).

Compendial expectations for sterilization and sterility assurance also exist. The appropriate documents for your region should be consulted when establishing the minimum validation requirements that should be met (Moldenhauer, 2014).

This list is not all-inclusive by any means. As such, you should be clear in your documents regarding the regulations applicable to you.

12.6 TYPES OF STERILIZATION PROCESSES

There are numerous types of sterilization processes: sterilizing filtration, radiation sterilization, gas sterilization, vaporized gas sterilization (decontamination), liquid phase sterilization, dry heat sterilization (and possibly depyrogenation), and moist heat sterilization. Sterilizing filtration, moist, and dry heat sterilization are most commonly used in pharmaceutical products, while gas sterilization and radiation sterilization are most commonly used in the medical device industry. Liquid phase sterilization (chemical sterilization) has not been widely used in the past in pharmaceuticals, but has increasing applicability with the need to sterilize cell cultures and tissue cultures in the biotechnology industry. This type of sterilization is also routinely used in the food industry, e.g., ozonated water (Moldenhauer, 2014).

12.6.1 STERILIZING FILTRATION FREQUENTLY MISNAMED AS ASEPTIC PROCESSING

Sterilizing filtration involves the filling of containers with ingredients that have been sterilized or are sterilized during the process (i.e., through a sterilizing filter). This is an extremely critical process as the filled container is not further processed in any other sterilization cycle. All the components are pre-sterilized and assembled in an aseptic environment using aseptic technique. This type of sterilization process is dependent upon the physical removal from the material to be sterilized not the destruction of the microorganisms present in the item. This section of the chapter specifically refers to a subset of aseptic processing, sterilizing filtration (Moldenhauer, 2014).

The filtration process can be used and validated to manufacture sterile products as defined by the USP < 1229 > *Sterilization of Compendial Articles* (USP 36 – NF31, 1229). This definition does not address the removal of viral contaminants. As such in biotechnology products that require absence of viral contaminants, additional steps must be taken to ensure they are removed from the item, these are frequently called viral exclusion and viral clearance studies (Moldenhauer, 2014).

There are several different factors that can affect the filtration process. When a filter is assessed for the ability to be used in a sterilization process, filter manufacturers frequently ask numerous questions that are taken into consideration in the filter validation like those aspects discussed in USP < 1229.4> (USP, 2013a; Moldenhauer, 2014):

- Type and number of microorganisms' present.
- Properties of the liquid being filtered, e.g., whether it is aqueous or oil-based, whether the entire liquid is soluble, the chemistry of the liquid, viscosity of the liquid, its surface tension, pH, osmolarity, ionic strength, and temperature.

- The design of the filter, e.g., whether it is a flat disk, a pleated filter, whether it has tortuous paths or non-tortuous paths, the area available for filtration, the nominal pore size, the thickness of the filter.
- Material used to manufacture the filter, e.g., mixed esters of cellulose, cellulose acetate, cellulose nitrate, polysulfone, polyvinylidene fluoride (PVDF).
- The process parameters for filtration, e.g., the temperature, flow rate, volumes to be filtered, the filtration time, the differential pressure. and pressure pulsations.

These types of parameters are so important, that the FDA requires that changes affecting many of these parameters be evaluated for their effect on the validation of the process (FDA, 2004; Moldenhauer, 2014).

The filter selected for the process is critical. As such, it is important to have a reliable supplier. Many companies choose to audit the filter supplier as part of their vendor audit program. During this review it is important to assess the methods used by the supplier to control production and the quality assurance systems in place to ensure that the filters are manufactured in accordance with the established specification. This should include their process to ensure the quality of the filter material (USP < 1229.4>, 2013a; Moldenhauer, 2014).

The end-user of the filter has many responsibilities in the sterilization process, one of which is to validate the effectiveness of the filter to sterilize the liquid processed through it. The user should define the allowable and validated parameters for the process and then establish controls to ensure that operations take place within the validated process. Some of the controls to be established are the requirements for filter integrity testing including both how and when it will be performed. There also should be requirements that specify what solution is evaluated in the test, e.g., the actual product or placebo or another solution. Additionally, they should have microbiological controls established to ensure that the bioburden level of the process does not exceed the capabilities of the filter (USP < 1229.4>, 2013a; 34Moldenhauer, 2014).

Specialized clean rooms are used for the sterilizing filtration process (ISO 5/ Grade A). Very tight standards exist for the particulate and viable microorganism levels that are allowed in these areas. Typically, the action level for viable microorganisms in an aseptic filling area environment is one colony forming unit (cfu) (FDA, 2004), although the European cGMP regulations in Annex 1 allow for an action level that averages to one cfu (EU GMPs, 2008) (Moldenhauer, 2014).

The FDA dramatically revised its guidance on aseptic filling and processing in 2004 (FDA, 2004). This document provides specific and clear guidance on the expectations for validation of sterilizing filtration and aseptic processes, as well as the sterilization and manufacturing processes used in support of the aseptic process. Since its issuance, the European Union's cGMPs (EU GMPs, 2008) and the Pharmaceutical Inspection Co-operation Scheme (PIC/s) have updated their requirements to be similar to the FDA document (PIC/s, 2011; Moldenhauer, 2014).

Validation of the process for sterilizing filtration of liquids is achieved by the successful performance of process simulation tests, also called media fills. Media fills are conducted after the completion of validation of the supporting systems, e.g., equipment sterilization, room and area cleaning and sanitization, qualification of disinfectants, environmental monitoring, validation of HVAC systems, gowning qualification, and so forth. An important pre-requisite is sufficient operator training to clearly understand acceptable aseptic behavior in the clean room. This is critical to maintain the aseptic area (Moldenhauer, 2014).

It can be difficult for clean room personnel to comprehend the impact of a quick movement in the room on the contamination level. One of the concerns is how slow should the movements be made to protect the environment. Some of the newer rapid microbiology technologies for environmental monitoring have the capability to measure viable microorganisms in real time. One of these technologies even has a webcam associated with the product, to record the actions taking place, especially in the event of a deviation being recorded. Allowing operators to mimic various actions they use and see/hear that it affects the counts and whether they stay within limits can be useful in training (Moldenhauer, 2014).

Designing the validation studies to perform requires careful thought and planning. One intent of the studies is to show that various interventions that occur in normal production can be performed maintaining the sterility of the solution filtered. One must also show that the process controls established are sufficient to produce a sterile liquid. The FDA's guidance describes the various parameters to consider in the validation study design (e.g., FDA 2004 and Moldenhauer 2014):

- Study Design – including evaluation of risk factors for contamination that could occur, worst case conditions, and assessing the process control.
- Frequency and Number of Runs – how often studies should be performed and the number of studies to perform.
- Duration of Runs – describes the model selected for the runs and how they are representative of the actual production run.
- Size of Runs – the number of units filled should be representative of production conditions. Typically, at least 5,000 units should be filled unless the routine production utilizes a smaller number of units. This should address batches manufacture over multiple shifts, or very high production volumes.
- Line Speed – the various line speeds used in production should be addressed, however only one line speed can be used in a specific media fill.
- Environmental Conditions – the study conditions should mimic actual production conditions. If possible, the conditions should be stressed, although not artificially created extremes.
- Media – the simulation should use a growth-promoting nutrient media.
- Incubation and Examination of Media-filled Units – the units should be incubated in a way to detect organisms that might be difficult to culture. Incubation temperatures should be within 20°–35°C, and within 2.5°C of the set-point temperature. The incubation time should be at least 14 days. During the incubation trained personnel should examine each unit for the presence of contamination.
- Interpretation of Results – In general no positive results can be obtained for fills less than 5,000 units. If the fill is greater than 5,000 units a single positive would result in an investigation and potentially another media fill (for units between 5,000 and 10,000 units), and two or more positives would require revalidation after the investigation.

The sterilizing filter used should have a pore size of 0.2 µm or smaller. It needs to be validated to ensure that it can remove microbiological contaminants (excluding virus removal) from the liquid. Challenge studies are typically performed with *Brevundimonas diminuta* (ATCC19146) as this organism is very small and a good challenge for this filter pore size. The validation should include a challenge of at least 10^7 microorganisms per cm^2 of filtration area (FDA, 2004; Moldenhauer, 2014).

Unlike many of the other types of sterilization processes available, you *cannot* calculate the sterility assurance level (SAL) of an aseptic filtration process. Many companies claim it has a SAL of 10^{-3}, but there are no valid calculations to do this. When we conduct process simulation runs (media fills) to validate the process we only get a snapshot in time of the contamination present in the process. This is different from a SAL calculation where you are determining the probability of a non-sterile unit in the process. Lack of contamination on one day does not give any mathematical probability of whether contamination will occur on a subsequent day (Moldenhauer, 2014).

Sterilizing aseptic filtration is the preferred method of sterilization for liquids that cannot withstand the rigors of other sterilization cycles. It does not add heat to the product and rarely, if ever, negatively affects the product stability (Moldenhauer, 2014).

12.6.2 CHEMICAL STERILIZATION METHODS – ALSO KNOWN AS LIQUID PHASE STERILIZATION

Chemical sterilization methods may be useful in situations where the item to be sterilized cannot withstand the heat associated with many other sterilization methods. Additionally, some items cannot be subjected to sterilizing filtration. Chemical sterilization methods are also useful in re-sterilizing medical devices, sterilizing in place lines within equipment, decontaminating equipment and drains, and the like. Chemical sterilization methods can be useful for these types of situations. Chemical sterilization involves subjecting the item to exposure with a chemical sterilant like the following (USP < 1229.6>, 2013b; Moldenhauer, 2014):

- Aldehydes: glutaraldehyde and formaldehyde. Note: Formaldehyde and glutaraldehyde are accepted more often in countries outside the USA.
- Acids: peracetic acid, nitric acid and sulfuric acid.
- Bases: sodium hydroxide, potassium hydroxide.
- Oxygenating Compounds: hydrogen peroxide, ozone (typically used as ozonated water), and chlorine dioxide. Note: for many food and cell culture operations ozonated water is used to achieve sterilization.
- Halides: sodium hypochlorite, chlorine.

Liquid phase sterilization is a type of chemical sterilization where the item is submersed or rinsed in the chemical solution. When these processes are conducted under the specified conditions, it is possible to eliminate bacterial and fungal contaminants (USP < 1229.6>, 2013b; ; Moldenhauer, 2014).

A key consideration in using chemical sterilants is whether the article to be sterilized is chemically compatible with the chemical sterilant. Many chemical sterilants can pose risks to the individuals working with them. As such, information on the safety issues associated with the sterilant is very important. In most cases, the vendor of the sterilant can provide this information. There are also many published articles on material compatibility with chemical sterilants (Moldenhauer, 2014).

An important consideration with using liquid phase sterilization is how the item will be removed and handled after being in the chemical sterilant. It is critical that it is not recontaminated, becoming unsuitable for use following the sterilization process. This can become extremely important when handling reusable medical devices, i.e., the maintenance of sterility.

The key factors to consider in the effectiveness of the sterilization cycle are: concentration of the sterilant and temperature although the pH, extent of mixing (if used), and soil (cells or cellular debris) may also be important. During validation it is common to use *Bacillus atrophaeus* ATCC 9372 or *Bacillus subtilis* ATCC 6633 as the biological indicator, since they are representative of worst case bioburden isolates. The indicators are directly inoculated upon the surface to be sterilized. Placement of the biological indicators should be determined by evaluating the most difficult areas for the sterilant to reach (USP < 1229.6>, 2013b; Moldenhauer, 2014).

Validation may be conducted using a half-cycle approach or the bracketing method. The premise of this approach is that a cycle is determined (exposure dwell time) that provides total kill of the biological indicator (starting population of 10^6). The exposure dwell time for routine production cycles is twice as much, resulting in a sterility assurance level or probability of a non-sterile unit of 10^{-6}. So, if you could validate a ten minute cycle to yield total kill of the biological indicator at 10^6 population, routine production would use a 20 minute cycle to provide a SAL of 10^{-6} (USP < 1229.6>, 2013b; Moldenhauer, 2014).

However, for most chemical sterilants there is a concern regarding whether the sterilant is effective for the entire sterilization cycle. They have modified the typical half-cycle approach to process the cycle for the half cycle, and then adding a second microbial challenge at the end of the half cycle to show that the biological indicator would again be inactivated in the second half of the cycle. This is a type of two-step validation and confirms that the chemical agent is effective in the second half of the full cycle. It is not a mandatory requirement to perform the testing in this way. Some only use the half-cycle approach and inoculate the item just at the beginning of the cycle (USP < 1229.6>, 2013b; Moldenhauer, 2014).

Another method that can be used for validation is the bracketing approach. In this method, the worst -case parameters for over-processing and under-processing are validated, allowing use of a cycle between these two sets of parameters. It is based upon the needs for the materials in the process and the bioburden. It is possible then for the user to determine the death rate for both extreme conditions tested. Short exposure times are common, due to the high inactivation rate of the sterilants. As such, one may have difficulty selecting cycles with recoverable biological indicators (USP < 1229.6>, 2013b; Moldenhauer, 2014).

The equipment used in these types of processes is subjected to the typical installation qualification and operational qualification. The loading of the equipment for the sterilization process is important. Chemical sterilants are surface sterilants, so the parts to be sterilized must come into contact with the sterilizing agent. This can be aided by use of mixing or recirculation during the sterilization process. For some of the water-based sterilants, the flow rate of the solution may also be an important parameter. It is common to define a maximum load per sterilizing chamber as it represents the maximum surface area to be sterilized (USP < 1229.6>, 2013b; Moldenhauer, 2014).

Successful validation is accomplished by performing sufficient replicates to show uniformity and reproducibility. During these cycles, parameters like biological indicator kill, sterilant concentration, exposure time, agitation or recirculation rates, and other key physical parameters (USP < 1229.6>, 2013b; Moldenhauer, 2014).

Unlike some other forms of sterilization, it is important to ensure that all the chemical sterilant is removed or inactivated following sterilization. This process must maintain the item in a sterilized manner. This should be evaluated from the completion of sterilization through placement into a sterile sealed container (USP < 1229.6, 2013b; Moldenhauer, 2014).

12.6.3 GAS STERILIZATION

Many types of instruments and medical devices cannot withstand the sterilization conditions associated with moist and dry heat sterilization. Gas sterilization is most commonly used with these types of equipment. Many gas sterilization processes use ethylene oxide (EtO), however other gases are being used today, e.g., chlorine dioxide), mixed oxides of nitrogen and ozone. There are some sterilants that exist in both a liquid and gas phase at the use temperatures, like hydrogen peroxide, peracetic acid, and paraformaldehyde. Some of these types of sterilants are discussed separately in the section called "Vapor Sterilization." (Agalloco, 2008; USP < 1229.7>, 2013c; Moldenhauer, 2014).

The key parameters of gas sterilization processes include: concentration, relative humidity, pressure, and temperature. Ethylene oxide (EtO) has the unique ability to penetrate through polymers, papers, and other materials. As such, it is frequently used for terminal sterilization of medical devices, even in their final packages. There are other gases that may be used for these kinds of processes (USP < 1229.7>, 2013c; Moldenhauer, 2014).

True gases are used allowing for single-point monitoring during operation to determine lethality. In some cases, more than one type of gas may be used concurrently (mixing). A difference between gas sterilization and other processes is that it does not condense during operation. The cycles must be developed to ensure sterility and maintaining the quality attributes of the product (USP < 1229.7>, 2013c; Moldenhauer, 2014).

Other important parameters for this type of cycle include: what are the immediate effects of the gas on the item being sterilized, the residual sterilants on the item, the by-products of the sterilants, and potential chemical reactions. Some chemical sterilants can be very corrosive, so this needs to be taken into consideration (USP < 1229.7>, 2013c; Moldenhauer, 2014).

12.6.3.1 Ethylene Oxide (EtO)

This type of process is used to sterilize items that are sensitive to temperatures greater than 60°C and/or they cannot be radiation sterilized. Some typical items

include plastics, options, and electrics (Wikipedia, 2013) In ethylene oxide sterilization, the strong alkylating agent destroys microorganisms – primarily the cell DNA.
This type of destruction follows first-order kinetics. It is dependent upon the concentration, humidity and temperature (USP < 1229.7>, 2013c and Moldenhauer, 2014).

A typical EtO cycle operates between 30° and 60°C, with relative humidity greater
than 30%, a gas concentration between 200 and 800 mg/L, and a typical cycle time
for at least three hours. EtO has good penetrability and is very effective, killing
viruses, bacteria and bacterial spores, and fungi. It has been shown to be compatible
with a variety of materials, even with more than one sterilization treatment. On the
negative side it is flammable, toxic and a carcinogen. It even has the potential to be
teratogenic (Wikipedia, 2013; Moldenhauer, 2014).

Typical sterilization cycles include preconditioning, rehumidification in the chamber, air removal, the gas exposure period, removal of gas from the sterilizer, and a
post-sterilization aeration to remove toxic residues. These cycles are widely used for
medical devices (Wikipedia, 2013; USP < 1229.7>, 2013c; Moldenhauer, 2014).

Ethylene oxide is different from heat-based cycles in that the gas is added at the
beginning of the cycle, with minimal additions of gas, i.e., only to maintain pressure. This gas can be explosive at concentrations greater than 3% volume in air
(USP < 1229.7>, 2013c) Validation and routine biological monitoring is conducted
using *Bacillus atrophaeus* (formerly called *Bacillus subtilis* variety niger and was
known as *Bacillus globigii*) (USP < 1229.7>, 2013c; Moldenhauer, 2014).

12.6.3.2 Ozone

Ozone is used in a variety of settings for food, medical devices, and pharmaceuticals. It is used to sterilize water and air. It is also used as a surface disinfectant
and sterilant. Unlike many disinfectants, it can oxidize most organic matter. On the
negative side it is toxic and unstable (i.e., it has a short half-life), so it needs to be
produced on site (Wikipedia, 2013; Moldenhauer, 2014).

Ozone is effective on a wide range of pathogens, including prions. It does not need
the use of hazardous chemicals to be effective. It is manufactured using medical
grade air. Following the use for sterilization, the waste material is converted back to
oxygen (Wikipedia, 2013; Moldenhauer, 2014).

Ozone is a strong oxidizing agent. It is manufactured by passing a stream of oxygen or air through a high-voltage electrical field. It has shown to be lethal in concentrations from 2% to 10% in the air. It works best when the relative humidity is
above 80%. Its degradation products are oxygen, in the presence of moisture and
metals. Unfortunately, it does not penetrate as well as EtO (USP < 1229.7>, 2013c;
Moldenhauer, 2014).

A typical sterilization process includes: humidification, injection, exposure, and
ventilation to remove the ozone following completion of the cycle. Biological challenges typically utilize *Geobacillus stearothermophilus* (USP < 1229.7>, 2013c;
Moldenhauer, 2014).

12.6.3.3 Nitrogen Dioxide (NO₂)

This type of gas can be used as a rapid and effective sterilant. It is effective against
many microorganisms including bacteria, viruses, and spores. This gas can be

used in an enclosed environment at room temperature and ambient pressure. Cells are inactivated by the degradation of DNA. It is effective at low concentrations of gas. It has a low boiling point of 21°C at sea level. As such, there is a high saturated vapor pressure at ambient temperature. With the low boiling point and the high saturated vapor pressure, condensation does not occur on the medical devices subjected to the sterilization process, and no post-sterilization aeration is required. It is compatible with many medical grade materials and adhesives. *Geobacillus stearothermophilus* is used as the biological indicator for this process (Wikipedia, 2013; Moldenhauer, 2014).

12.6.3.4 Chlorine Dioxide

Another gas used for sterilization is chlorine dioxide. This type of gas is metastable meaning that it is stable, provided it is subjected to no more than small disturbances. Due to the difficulty in maintaining stability, it must be generated when needed for use. It is not a carcinogen nor is it flammable. It works at ambient conditions, but does not penetrate as well as EtO (USP < 1229.7>, 2013c; Moldenhauer, 2014).

"Chlorine dioxide is a chemical compound with the formula ClO_2. This yellowish-green gas crystallizes as bright orange crystals at −59°C. As one of several oxides of chlorine, it is a potent and useful oxidizing agent used in water treatment and in bleaching" (Wikipedia, 2018).

Typical sterilization cycles include: preconditioning, conditioning dwell period, charge, exposure, and aeration. The biological indicator of choice is *Bacillus atrophaeus* (USP < 1229.7>, 2013c; Moldenhauer, 2014).

Eylath et al. (2003) describes the successful use of this technology when sterilizing an aseptic filling line isolator. The authors reported that the chlorine dioxide distribution was excellent in this study, with variability throughout the isolator and its associated ducts measured at less than 0.2 mg/L at an exposure concentration of 5 mg/L.

Lowe et al. (2013) found gaseous ClO_2 effective for sterilization in hospital rooms, when tested against common contaminants for nosocomial infections. In this study, concentrations of ClO_2 up to 385 ppm were safely maintained in a hospital room with enhanced environmental controls.

12.6.3.5 Validating Gas Sterilization Processes

The most common method of validation is the half-cycle approach. It is a variety of an overkill approach. In this cycle type, you determine what is required to kill all the biological indicators (10^6 spores) for validation and routinely double the cycle for routine production, corresponding to a PNSU of 10^{-6}. There have been other approaches to validation developed, including the Gillis and Mosley Parametric Evaluation and a Bracketing Approach (USP < 1229.7>, 2013c; Moldenhauer, 2014).

- Equipment qualification is conducted like other sterilization equipment. It should include the requirements for all phases of sterilization from the pre-humidification steps through any post cycle aeration or other phases. Completion of this qualification should show that the equipment is installed and operating as intended.

- Empty Chamber Distribution Study: Many still perform this type of study to show that the methods used for introduction of gas and humidity is consistent and uniform. It may also provide useful information on the routine monitoring positions to use. No biological indicators are utilized (USP < 1229.7>, 2013c; Moldenhauer, 2014).
- Component and Load Mapping: This type of study is typically not included for gas sterilization, as the conduct of the study would alter the gas and humidity parameters. Biological indicators (passive) or control devices may be placed within load items that are expected to be hardest for gas and humidity penetration to evaluate these parameters (USP < 1229.7>, 2013c; Moldenhauer, 2014).
- Biological indicators: *Bacillus atrophaeus* (ATCC 9372) is used for all but ozone sterilization. For ozone *Geobacillus stearothermophilus* (ATCC 12980 or 7953) is the indicator of choice (USP < 1229.7>, 2013c; Moldenhauer, 2014).
- Process Confirmation – Microbiological Challenge Studies: Combination studies are performed using physical, chemical, and microbiological challenges concurrently. The sensors are placed in the chamber, while the biological challenges are located within the load items. Replicate studies are required to show reproducibility and efficacy (USP < 1229.7>, 2013c; Moldenhauer, 2014).
- Routine Process Control: Once validated, care should be taken to maintain the sterilizer in a qualified condition. This includes things like: change control, establishment of procedures for operation and control, performing periodic evaluations of performance, routine calibration, and the like.

12.6.3.6 Vapor Sterilization

Various types of vapor can be used for sterilization including hydrogen peroxide, formaldehyde (not widely accepted for use in the USA, but is used in the EU), and peracetic acid. Some also choose to vaporize ozone gas. In many cases they are used and claimed for decontamination rather than sterilization. The chemical vapors have limited volatility at room temperature in air. Raising the temperature of the inlet stream is used for hydrogen peroxide and formaldehyde to increase the efficiency. It is mixed at temperatures above the boiling point to and the vapor and air are mixed. The hot "mixed" air is mixed further in the sterilizer chamber. Unfortunately, as the hot air contacts with the colder surfaces in the chamber, condensation occurs. Aggressive mixing is needed in the vessel to achieve uniformity. The system lends itself to high relative humidity, but care must be taken to achieve uniform temperature ranges across the chamber in order to get uniform humidity. Some variation always occurs, with the inlet stream being very hot. It is also likely to obtain differences in concentration on the surface for water and the vapor. Minimal penetration exists for the vapors. Use of vapors for sterilization is intrinsically more difficult than true gas sterilization processes (Agalloco, 2008; Moldenhauer, 2014).

12.6.3.6.1 Hydrogen Peroxide (H₂O₂)

In a hydrogen peroxide cycle, the first step is to remove the humidity from the chamber. This is accomplished using low humidity air circulation, followed by a brief conditioning to increase the hydrogen peroxide concentration rapidly. The "exposure dwell period" is next. During this period the hydrogen peroxide concentration is maintained by continuously addition or periodic injections. Following exposure, the aeration phase takes place using low humidity air to re-evaporate the hydrogen peroxide from the surfaces (Agalloco, 2008; Moldenhauer, 2014).

Hydrogen peroxide is a strong oxidizing agent, which makes it effective against a wide range of pathogens. It can be dangerous as concentrations higher than 10% w/w. The cycle time for hydrogen peroxide is much lower than for EtO. The strong oxidizing power of hydrogen peroxide can also be a negative, as it can have issues with material compatibility. According to the information for the Sterrad system, paper products cannot be sterilized with this method due to cellulosics, a process where all of the hydrogen peroxide is absorbed by the paper product. Additionally, this vapor does not have the penetrating power of EtO (Wikipedia, 2013; Moldenhauer, 2014).

There are safety concerns to personnel that also must be addressed with the use of hydrogen peroxide. The vapor is frequently used to sterilize large areas and sealed areas like clean rooms and the inside of aircraft (Wikipedia, 2013; Moldenhauer, 2014).

12.6.3.6.2   Peracetic Acid

Sterilization is achieved by misting this product and water throughout the chamber. Wetted surfaces are not sterilized. This necessitates the use of care in arranging the items in the load and the injection site. The items are held for a defined period and the liquid is evaporated using how humidity air. It can be an effective surface sterilants (Agalloco, 2008; Moldenhauer, 2014).

12.6.3.6.3   Validating Vapor Sterilization Processes

In vapor sterilization it is not as easy to measure concentration, humidity, and temperature (though not as important a parameter) as in gas sterilization. The key is to have reproducible attainment of the combined parameters. Cycles are performed to show reproducibility using a resistant biological indicator. One can use fraction negative cycles to show the resistance of the biological indicator to the process (Agalloco, 2008; Moldenhauer, 2014).

Most use the half-cycle approach for qualification of these processes. The cycle is set at eight to nine times the D-value, which allows for an appropriate safety factor to be established. The routine cycle is twice this length. All biological indicators must be inactivated (Agalloco, 2008; Moldenhauer, 2014).

12.6.3.7   Radiation Sterilization

There are a variety of radiation processes that can be used, but most utilize gamma rays or electron beams. X-rays and ultraviolet light are also used. The effect of the radiation on the items being sterilized should be assessed. The radiation is used to destroy the microorganisms present. Radiation sterilization has several advantages including: simplicity, lack of mechanical complexity, reproducibility, and overall efficiency (USP < 1229.10>, 2013e; Moldenhauer, 2014).

The key concept of the sterilization process is the amount of radiation (dose) that is absorbed by the item. This dose can be precisely measured. ISO 11137-1 (sterilization of health care products) describes the various ways to determine the

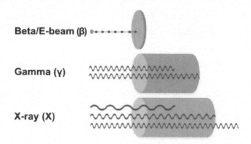

FIGURE 12.1 Penetration Differences for Different Types of Radiation Figure Courtesy of Wikipedia (Dethierp, 2013).

dose that should be used. They have methods called, Method 1, Method 2A, Method 2B, and Method VDmax. These methods have different testing approaches and the number of times to use for testing. These differences are based upon the assumptions regarding bioburden. Biological indicators are not used since accurate correlations exist between the measurement of the dose and the destruction of a variety of microbes. The measurement process – dosimetry – is used to assess the lethality achieved in the process. It is measured in kGy. It is directly related to the microbial lethal effects due to radiation, similar to the F_0 calculation in moist heat sterilization. Dosimeters can be used on the items being sterilized to assess process performance (USP < 1229.10>, 2013e; Moldenhauer, 2014) (Figures 12.1 and 12.2).

12.6.3.8 Gamma Sterilization

Gamma sterilization is conducted in a specialty facility that is tightly controlled. In this facility, the items to be sterilized are subjected to radiation from Cobalt 60 (Co60). This type of radiation allows for a uniform dose to be delivered. Gamma rays are emitted from the Co60 during the decay process where it becomes Ni60. This specific isotope has a half-life of 5.25, or it loses about 12% of its radioactivity each year. Due to this decay process, the cycle requires regular adjustment to

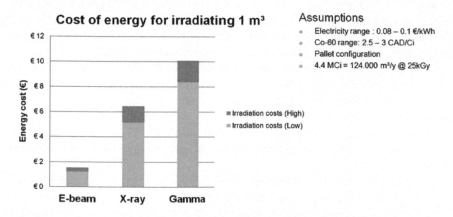

FIGURE 12.2 Cost of Irradiation Using Different Processes Figure courtesy of Wikipedia (Dethierp, 2013).

ensure that the required dose is delivered. This may necessitate adding additional Co60 in the process to maintain the appropriate dose (USP < 1229.10>, 2013e; Moldenhauer, 2014).

The items being sterilized by irradiation do not become radioactive (Wikipedia, 2013) However, the radiation may affect the properties of the material (Bharati et al., 2009; Moldenhauer, 2014)

12.6.3.8.1   X-Ray Sterilization

Bremsstrahlung or high-energy (high power) X-rays are used in medical device processes for sterilization. They are useful since large packages and pallet loads can be sterilized using this technology. The ability to penetrate the package is very good when using loads of low-density packages. It has good dose uniformity ratios (Wikipedia, 2013; Moldenhauer, 2014).

This type of sterilization is an electricity-based process. Neither chemical nor radioactive material is required. An X-ray machine is used to generate the X-rays. Fortunately, this machine can be turned on when in use and turned off when not in use. It also does not require the various protections needed for other types of radiation sterilization, e.g., shielding (Wikipedia, 2013; Moldenhauer, 2014).

X-rays are a result of colliding accelerated electrons with a dense material called the target. Materials like tantalum and tungsten may be used. The conversion requires a higher level of electrical energy than some other systems (Wikipedia, 2013; Moldenhauer, 2014).

The photons generated in this type of process are highly penetrative. The materials to be sterilized are scanned with X-ray photons. If the systems are maintained appropriately, a constant sterilization does is delivered (USP < 1229.10>, 2013e; Moldenhauer, 2014).

12.6.3.8.2   Electron-Beam (E-Beam) Sterilization

This type of sterilization provides a significantly higher dose rating than gamma or X-rays. As such, a lower exposure time is required, which in turn reduces the potential for product degradation. Electron beams do not have the penetrative efficiency of gamma or X-rays. Shielding, typically concrete, is used to protect the surrounding environment and personnel (Wikipedia, 2013; Moldenhauer, 2014).

Sterilizers for this technology are available for both batch and continuous processes. Items to be sterilized are scanned with the electron beam within a defined radiation field. When appropriately controlled and operated, the systems deliver a constant dose over time. The higher dose rate and the absence of a local radioactive source make this type of sterilization attractive. The systems themselves come in small sizes that may be operated by the end-user (USP < 1229.10>, 2013e; Moldenhauer, 2014).

Care must be taken in developing the sterilization cycles as the penetration is much lower than obtained with photons. This higher dose rate can also lead to the items experiencing higher temperatures than in a gamma cycle. Dose mapping is very important to guarantee that items are properly sterilized (USP < 1229.10>, 2013e; Moldenhauer, 2014).

12.6.3.8.3 Validating Radiation Sterilization Processes

A key consideration in the development of a radiation sterilization cycle is the effective radiation dose for the times to be sterilized, while showing that this dose does not adversely affect the item's key quality attributes. Both the minimum and maximum allowable dose should not cause adverse effects to the item (USP < 1229.10>, 2013e; Moldenhauer, 2014).

ISO standards identify various types of dose setting methods, Method 1, Method 2A, Method 2B, and Method VDmax. Selecting the right method to use is dependent upon the production batch size, the bioburden present, and the sensitivity of the item's sensitivity to the type of radiation used (USP < 1229.10>, 2013e; Moldenhauer, 2014).

- Radiation Dose: As the ionizing radiation penetrates an object, it deposits energy. The energy that is absorbed from radiation exposure is called a dose.
- Dose Setting: Using Method 1, the dose is compared to the radiation resistance of the bioburden. Typical D-value or resistance studies are not determined, but rather a standard radiation resistance is used from the literature. The belief is that the standard resistance is a greater challenge than the routine bioburden. The site performs a verification dose study and determines the appropriate dose from a table. This is similar to the VDmax method, requiring bioburden and dose verification testing, but is dependent upon low bioburden in the item to be sterilized. The assumption is < 1000 cfu for a 25 kGy sterilization dose and 0.1 – 1.5 cfus per item for a 15 kGy sterilization dose. Method 2 is more complex. It uses a series of incremental dose exposures to establish a dose. The intent is that one sample out of 100 if treated with that dose will be non-sterile. This dose determination process provides a way to determine the dose. The intent is to determine the dose that will result in one sample out of 100 non-sterile samples (USP < 1229.10>, 2013e; Moldenhauer, 2014).
- Compatibility of Materials: Following the determination of the required dose, a corresponding maximum dose is established. This dose represents the highest dose that is likely to be seen in a sterilization cycle, adding a safety factor, and based upon the effects on the materials in the item both immediate and long term (USP < 1229.10>, 2013e; Moldenhauer, 2014).
- Dose Verification: During cycle development and dose setting the methods are dependent upon the bioburden approach. Cycle efficacy depends upon appropriate control of pre-sterilization bioburden and periodic monitoring of the process' effect on bioburden. Dose setting is based upon the natural resistance of the bioburden and extrapolates to ensure a PNSU of 1×10^{-6}.
- Equipment Qualification: Initial qualification and periodic requalification studies are performed to ensure appropriate equipment performance. The key parameters in qualification differ based upon the type of sterilization process. For gamma sterilization, key parameters are equipment controls and the parameters for the system's capability. E-beam and X-ray sterilization utilize controls for scan speed, source intensity, and system timers (USP < 1229.10>, 2013e; Moldenhauer, 2014).

- Empty Chamber Dose Mapping: This type of study, while not required provides a useful baseline of performance (USP < 1229.10>, 2013e; Moldenhauer, 2014).
- Load Mapping: The purpose of this study is to determine the appropriate arrangement of items in the load that minimizes the dose variation across items. Several dosimeters are used in both internal and external positions. This type of study can also be used to determine the effects of the maximum sterilization dose.
- Biological Indicators: The use of biological indicators is contraindicated as the dosimeters are more reliable, reproducible, and robust (USP < 1229.10>, 2013e; Moldenhauer, 2014).
- Dosimetry: Cycle development and qualification requires the use of periodically calibrated dosimeters (USP < 1229.10>, 2013e).
- Process Confirmation: Replicate studies are performed to show reproducible acceptable lethality, based upon the results from the dosimeters. They should be strategically placed across the material in the process (USP < 1229.10>, 2013e; Moldenhauer, 2014).
- Routine Process Control: Controls must be established to ensure that the systems are maintained and controlled within the validated sterilization parameters.

12.6.3.9   Moist Heat Sterilization

Before addressing the topic of moist heat sterilization, it is important to differentiate between moist and dry heat. Moist heat sterilization is defined as a sterilization process that uses steam under pressure, as is conducted in an autoclave. The steam is considered saturated when the steam and the water are in equilibrium. A closed container of water, when heated to temperatures in excess of 100°C, will demonstrate an increase in the steam pressure. As the temperature rises, so does the pressure. There are steam tables that can be utilized to show the relationship between temperature and pressure. When the steam is saturated, raising the pressure using external means will result in the steam starting to condense back into water. Superheated steam is defined as steam whose temperature, at a given pressure, is higher than that indicated by the equilibration curve for the vaporization of water. The thermal energy (heat) delivered by different heating media using different types of moist heat sterilization processes like saturated steam, air/steam mixtures, or superheated water, at the same temperature is significantly different (PDA Technical Report Number 1, 2007; Moldenhauer, 2013 and 2014).

With moist heat sterilization, the microorganisms present are destroyed by coagulating and denaturing the cell's enzymes and structural proteins. Typical sterilization cycles require that the exposure time be at 121°C in the range of 15 to 30 minutes for the spores most resistant to the sterilization process. These processes can be performed at other temperatures that yield equivalent lethality to those at a specified reference temperature (Moldenhauer, 2013 and 2014).

Moist heat sterilization processes are used to sterilize equipment in support of the sterile processing of pharmaceutical products, cleaning supplies used in some clean room operations, primary packaging materials, terminal sterilization of liquid-filled containers, and so forth (Moldenhauer, 2013 and 2014).

Dry heat sterilization refers to the use of hot air that is free of water vapor, or has very little water vapor. In this type of process, the moisture present has little effect on the sterilization process. Dry heat sterilization has been used for many years. It is believed to be less complicated than moist heat sterilization. Sterilization is achieved by using much higher temperatures for much longer time periods. Pharmaceuticals often use temperatures exceeding 250°C, however some guidance indicates that one may use temperatures greater than 160°C. Dry heat kills microorganisms by destructive oxidation of essential cell constituents. There are bacterial spores that are resistant to dry heat sterilization although they may not be used in the validation of these processes. Frequently endotoxin challenges are conducted concurrently with the validation of these cycles. If used appropriately, the endotoxin challenges eliminate the need to use biological indicators are since the endotoxin challenge is more severe than the resistance of the biological indicator. Dry heat sterilization processes are used for glassware, and some equipment that can withstand the higher temperatures for the prolonged periods of time required (Moldenhauer, 2013 and 2014).

Use of a steam sterilizer does not ensure that all parts of the load are subjected to moist heat. It isn't sufficient to supply moist heat (steam) into the sterilizer. In steam sterilization, the moist heat must come into contact with the items being sterilized. Some items make it difficult or impossible for all of the air to be removed from them as well as allowing steam to penetrate. In these situations, they may be achieving sterilization through dry heat only. Some examples include: filter housings, long tubing, tightly closed containers. It is important to ensure that the items being sterilized are coming into contact with the sterilizing media that you intend to use (Moldenhauer, 2013 and 2014).

12.6.3.9.1   Sterilizer Configurations

For moist heat, sterilizers there are both batch configurations and continuous sterilizers available. Few pharmaceutical companies choose to use continuous sterilizers. However, they are often used in the food industry. Most pharmaceutical sterilizers used are operated as a batch unit, i.e., material is moved to the sterilizer, processed in the sterilizer, and following sterilization is moved to the next production step. Batch sterilizers are available in a variety of sizes from bench top sized to laboratory sized, to units that handle two or more sterilizer trucks or pallets of loads. Some sterilizers are the size of railroad cars (Moldenhauer, 2013 and 2014).

Sterilizers can be configured to be specific for one type of sterilization process or may be able to perform more than one type of sterilization process (multi-function sterilizers). Some of the typical sterilization processes available are: saturated steam, steam-air mixtures, air overpressure cycles, and those which use superheated water (e.g., water-spray, raining water, water immersion, and rotary sterilization cycles) (PDA Technical Report Number 1, 2007; Moldenhauer, 2014).

PDA's Technical Report Number 1 (2007) has further divided moist heat sterilization cycles into those used for porous (and hard goods) loads and those used for liquid loads. In this document they have defined porous loads as "loads of materials for which the contaminant microbial populations are inactivated through direct contact with the steam supplied to the sterilizer. For porous loads heat transfer is through steam condensing directly on items being processed, unlike fluid loads where steam acts principally as an agent for heat transfer." Some examples of porous loads are those used to sterilize filter cartridges, garments, stoppers, tubing, and so forth. This same document defines liquid loads as "Liquid filled container loads within the production setting are usually homogeneous, comprised of containers of a single size, single fill volume, and derived from a single lot. Some examples of liquid loads are liquid-filled vials and syringes. Liquid load cycles are developed and validated frequently using the Product Specific Approach though the overkill method may also be used." (PDA Technical Report Number 1, 2007; Moldenhauer, 2013) The USP in its < 1229 > series of sterilization documents has classified them as Steam Sterilization by Direct Contact and Moist Heat Sterilization of Aqueous Liquids (USP < 1229>, 2012a; Moldenhauer, 2014).

12.6.3.9.2   Determining Worst Case Conditions

Overkill cycles deliver the most heat to the product and have the highest safety factor of sterility assurance. For products, they can also have the highest level of impact on the product stability. Typically, they are routinely used for sterilization of porous loads, hard goods, and some terminal sterilization activities, when the item is not heat sensitive. The worst-case overkill cycle may be determined by lowering the sterilizing temperature by 1°C, or more and reducing the exposure time by a few minutes from the set-point conditions, i.e., either at the minimum allowable conditions or below these conditions (sub-lethal). Alternatively, if one uses a load probe they can execute the study with a lower F_0 than the values routinely allowed. Following the approach used in gaseous sterilization some use the *half-cycle* approach for validation, where the sterilization time used in the performance qualification is doubled for the routine production cycle. This approach is only useful if the excessive heat will not affect the product. The cycles developed for an overkill process are expected to totally destroy the biological indicator challenge utilized (Agalloco, 2008; Moldenhauer 2013 and 2014).

Product-specific cycles are used most often for terminal sterilization of products. In the USP chapter for moist heat sterilization of liquids, these types of cycles are described as bioburden based approaches or biological indicator-bioburden-based approaches (USP < 1229.2>, 2012b). Validation is performed at the minimum conditions allowed for acceptable release of the product. These requirements may require total destruction of the biological indicator or have a requirement for a specific biological indicator log reduction or $F_{Biological}$. Additionally, there are requirements established for the maximum heat delivered to the product, typically as either specified upper time/temperature requirements and/or a provision for the maximum allowable F_0 (the maximum allowable lethality delivered to the product). Resistant bioburden is an integral part in determining the lethality required. Therefore, these types of cycles require an ongoing, vigilant evaluation of bioburden recovered in the plant, including an assessment of its heat resistance (Moldenhauer, 2013) Note: In the USP monograph (USP < 1229.2>, 2013b) maximum F_0 is only required for moist heat sterilization of liquids (Moldenhauer, 2014).

12.6.3.9.3   Load Configurations

The load size and arrangement is also an important factor in the efficacy of the sterilization cycle. In porous load sterilization, it is important that the items be placed on the sterilizer carts or pallets in such a way that they do not adversely affect the sterilization of other items in the load, e.g., not dripping condensate from one item onto another item. It is common to have a fixed loading pattern, which identifies the specific locations where items are to be placed. Heavier items are placed on the bottom of the load. Fixed loading patterns are also used for liquid loads. The containers may be placed into trays or on sterilizer carts in a defined arrangement. It is common to have detailed drawings or photographs which clearly delineate the loading arrangements to be used (Moldenhauer, 2013 and 2014).

Following sterilization, items may be removed and transported to other areas for use or may not be used immediately, provisions are made to ensure that the item sterilized maintains its sterile state. This may include wrapping the item with sterilizer wrap or placing it into sterilizer bags or pouches. When this is done, the methods should be established so that the wrapping or pouching process does not adversely affect the air removal or steam penetration (Moldenhauer, 2013 and 2014).

During cycle development, one should determine which items heat-up faster than others and which are the slowest to heat-up. Within specific items, studies are performed to evaluate the hardest-to-heat area of the item, which is where the thermocouples are placed. This may be accomplished placing multiple probes or biological indicators into the item. If probes are used, the heating characteristics of the item are mapped, and the lowest probe value is where the thermocouples are placed in subsequent studies. Alternatively, biological indicators may be used to assess where the lowest level of kill is achieved and then this is the probing location. With biological indicators it is common to use sub-lethal cycles to ensure growth of the indicators after sterilization (Moldenhauer, 2014).

You may validate both the minimum and maximum allowable loading configuration. However, the PDA's Technical Report Number 1 (2007) indicates that neither of these configurations may be the worst case (Moldenhauer, 2013 and 2014).

12.6.3.9.4   Cycle Monitoring

Routine monitoring parameters for moist heat sterilization cycles include: come-up time, exposure time and temperature, cooling time or final temperature, water temperature (for superheated water cycles), fan speed (for fan cycles), pressure, time at which air is added to the cycle (air overpressure), and so forth (Moldenhauer, 2013 and 2014).

12.6.3.9.4.1   Sterilization and How Microorganisms Die   A significant amount of research has been conducted studying the kinetics of microbial death. They found that the process of destroying or sterilizing the cells occurs at a defined and consistent rate that is dependent upon the variables that affect the reaction rate, as shown in Figure 12.3. The D-value is determined by plotting the number of viable cells (survivors) on the y-axis and the exposure time on the x-axis. A best-fit line is drawn through the points. The line can be reviewed graphically to determine the time it takes to reduce the microbial population by one log at a specified set of sterilization conditions (Agalloco, 2008; Moldenhauer, 2014). However, today most people just use the calculator to determine the D-value using the equations from PDA Technical Report Number 1 (2007).

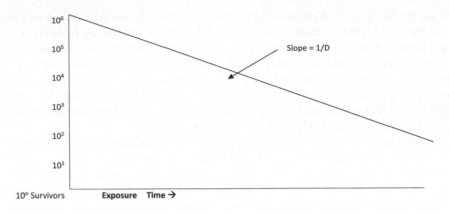

FIGURE 12.3 Microorganisms Die in a Logarithmic Fashion at a Defined Set of Parameters.

This relative relationship has led to the development of a number of calculations that can be used to model the microbial destruction and the probability of sterility associated with a sterilization cycle.

One of the most effective types of sterilization is moist heat (steam) under pressure. To use this methodology, the item to be sterilized must be able to withstand heat and moisture without damage. It is reported that most microbes grow in the range of −50°C to 80°C, although some form spores at temperatures outside of these ranges (DeSantis, 2008; Moldenhauer, 2013 and 2014).

Sterilization applications utilize the understanding of how microorganisms die, to predict the probability of a survivor in a sterilization process. This is expressed as PNSU or the probability of a non-sterile unit. For moist heat sterilization the expected PNSU is less than 10^{-6}, which means that there is no more than a one in a million probability of a non-sterile unit. Not all sterilization processes predict the probability of non-sterility. For example, an aseptic process validation measures the rate of contamination present at the time the process simulation test was performed but does not provide a probabilistic measure of the sterility assurance (Moldenhauer, 2013 and 2014).

Copious information is available that indicates that microbial death can be described as a first-order chemical reaction. This implies that the death is a single molecule reaction, probably because of a denaturization of a specific critical molecule in the cell (DeSantis, 2008; Moldenhauer, 2014).

12.6.3.9.4.2 Biological Indicators Some types of bacteria (Gram-positive rods) can form structures that are resistant to adverse conditions called spores as a defensive survival method. These are different from fungal spores (mold spores) that are manufactured as reproductive bodies. The genus and species of bacteria resistant to a specific sterilization process may be different across sterilization processes. Additionally, the same bacterial spore may have different levels of resistance to varying sterilization processes. The level of resistance to a sterilization process is expressed as the D-value. D-values are specific for a sterilization medium and a specific temperature. The D-value is defined as the amount of time in minutes that are required at a specific reference temperature to reduce the microbial population by one log. The higher the D-value at a specific set of sterilizing conditions, the more resistant the organism is to the sterilization process (Moldenhauer, 2013 and 2014).

12.6.3.9.4.3 D-values   *Geobacillus stearothermophilus* spores ($D_T \sim 1.5$–6.0 minutes in various parenteral solutions) are considered one of the most resistant spores for moist heat sterilization. As such, many regulatory documents specify the use of these spores in the validation of moist heat sterilization cycles. Some other organisms have been identified that have sufficient resistance to be appropriate challenges for validation of moist heat sterilization cycles include: *Bacillus subtilis* 5230 ($D_T \sim 0.5$ minute in 0.9% Saline), *Bacillus smithii* (formerly *Bacillus coagulans*, FRR B666) ($D_T \sim 1.5$ minute in sterile water), and *Clostridium sporogenes* ATCC 7955 ($D_T \sim 0.3$–7.0 minutes in various parenteral solutions) (Sadowski, 2009; Moldenhauer, 2011) It is important to know the regulatory expectations in your country when selecting the appropriate biological indicator challenge to use (Moldenhauer, 2013 and 2014).

A variety of spores are also available for dry heat sterilization. Typically, spores of *Bacillus subtilis* have been used. Some have successfully used *Geobacilllus stearothermophilus*. Typically, the most resistant of spores will have a D-value of six to ten minutes at 170°C. If the cycle is used to depyrogenate and is run at a much higher temperature, the microbial D-values may be only a few seconds (Pharmaceutical Validation, 2011; Moldenhauer, 2013 and 2014).

Selection of the biological indicator to use includes consideration of many things including: an organism that is not pathogenic; an organism that is easy to cultivate; an organism that can be cleaned, harvested, and grown with relative ease; an organism more resistant to the sterilization process than the items being sterilized; an organism which is stable; an organism which is not inhibited by the items it will be used to test; and an organism which provides reproducible results when tested at a specific temperature (Sadowski, 2009; Moldenhauer, 2013 and 2014).

For moist heat sterilization cycles, the biological indicator to be used in the process is based upon the sterilization cycle-design model (approach) used. Most companies using an overkill model choose to use *Geobacillus stearothermophilus*. When product-based models are used, the other acceptable biological indicators are frequently used (Sadowski, 2009; Moldenhauer, 2013 and 2014).

12.6.3.9.4.4 z-values   Another important term when using biological indicators is the z-value. This term refers to the temperature dependence on the D-value. It represents the number of degrees of temperature that are required to achieve a ten-fold change in the D-value. For example, if the z-value is 10°C, changing the sterilizing temperature from 120° to 130°C will yield a ten-fold change in the D-value. As such, a much shorter sterilization time will be required at the higher temperature. The z-value tends to be constant across a broader range of temperatures. *Geobacillus stearothermophilus* spores have a typical z-value of 10°C for temperatures between 100° to 135°C. *Bacillus subtilis* spores used for dry heat have a typical z-value of 20°C in the range of 150° to 190°C. Dry heat cycles used to concurrently depyrogenate using temperatures of 225° to 300°C, the z-values used are between 45° to 53°C (Agalloco, 2008; Moldenhauer, 2013 and 2014).

12.6.3.9.4.5　F-value　The F-value or thermal death time is used along with the temperature data and z-value to estimate the lethality for moist and dry heat sterilization cycles (Agalloco, 2008) It is the time in minutes required to deliver a sterilization cycle equivalent to that of the reference temperature T. For most moist heat sterilization cycles the reference temperature is 121°C and for dry heat sterilization cycles it may be 160° or 250°C (Moldenhauer, 2013 and 2014).

The reference temperature benchmarks the cycle in terms of the heat delivered at the specified temperature. The F-value is specific for a defined reference temperature. Equation 12.1 provides the equation for the F-value (PDA, 2007; DeSantis, 2008; Moldenhauer, 2013 and 2014).

$$F = \int 10^{(T_0 - T\text{ref}/Z)} dt \qquad (12.1)$$

This formula approximates to:

$$F = \sum 10^{(T_0 - T\text{ref}/Z)} \Delta t \qquad (12.2)$$

where,

T_0 = Temperature within the item being heated
T_{ref} = Reference temperature
Z = z-value of the challenge organism
dt = the change in time (minutes)
Δt = he chosen time interval (minutes)

For moist heat sterilization, when the reference temperature is 121.1°C and the z-value is 10°C, the F-value is called F_0. For dry heat sterilization, many use the term F_H where the reference temperature is dependent upon whether the cycle is used for sterilization or depyrogenation. Some companies use a F_P designation for depyrogenation (Moldenhauer, 2014).

Figure 12.4 provides an example of a microbial survivor curve for moist heat sterilization. Although this is example is for moist heat, similar curves can be performed for dry heat. In this figure, the starting population of resistant microorganisms, N_0 is 10^6. The D-value at the specified reference temperature is 2.5 minutes. The desired level for the probability of a non-sterile unit is 10^{-6}. The desired probability of survivors in this graph is designated as N_F, or the final population (PDA Technical Report Number 1, 2007; Moldenhauer, 2013 and 2014).

The microbial survival curve model is representative of first-order kinetics, i.e., the death kinetics of single-celled spores. While this model may not be representative all of the different types of challenge systems, this is still the best model available. To properly use this model in microbial destruction calculations it is important that the challenge organism is in a homogeneous culture and that the constant lethal stress or

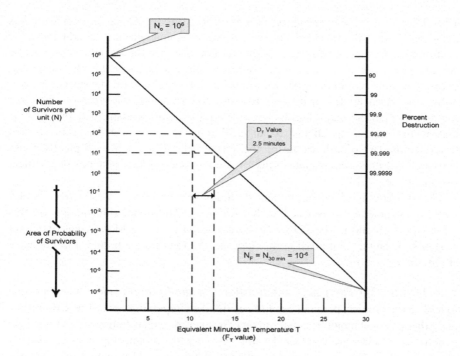

FIGURE 12.4   Microbial Survivor Curve.

the equivalent lethal stress is applied to the challenge (PDA, 2007; Moldenhauer, 2013 and 2014).

12.6.3.9.4.6   Probability of a Non-Sterile Unit (PNSU)   The probability of a nonsterile unit calculation is used to determine the likelihood of obtaining a non-sterile unit at the end of the sterilization cycle. Generally, it is accepted that an acceptable probability is one in a million, or 10^{-6} for sterilization. Some assume this is a synonymous term with sterility assurance level (SAL). The exponent for the SAL should be a positive number rather than the negative exponent in a PNSU value. Many prefer the term PNSU since the values of the exponents are not ambiguous. The PNSU can be calculated by solving for B, using Equation 12.3 (Agalloco, 2008; Moldenhauer, 2013 and 2014):

$$\text{Log}_{10}\, B = \text{Log}_{10}\, A - \left(F_0 \,/\, D_{121} \right) \tag{12.3}$$

where,
B = Probability of a Non-Sterile Unit
A = Number of Pre-sterilization Bioburden Microorganisms
F_0 = The minimum F_0 observed in the cycle
D_{121} = The D-value of the bioburden microorganism at the reference temperature
     of 121°C
Note: For cycles using other F-values or D-values, the values would be substituted
     for F_0 and D_{121} (Moldenhauer, 2014).

12.6.3.9.4.7   Commissioning or Engineering Studies   Once the sterilizer has been installed at the intended location, there are some activities conducted prior to initiating the formal validation of the system. Some of the activities that may be conducted include: cleaning, addition of lubricants, and so forth. It is also beneficial to execute some runs of the sterilizer to take a "look-see" on how the system is operating. The engineers frequently use this time to ensure that the system is sequencing as expected, no major alarms occur, and a general assessment if the systems appears to be operating reliably so that validation can commence. This is performed to reduce the risk of failures during the actual validation process. Typically, these activities fall under the responsibility of the engineering/maintenance department (Moldenhauer, 2013).

Commissioning of the equipment includes verifying that the sterilizer is performing sufficiently to proceed with validation. Additional information on this topic can be found in the PDA's Technical Report No. 48 Moist Heat Sterilizer Systems: Design, Commissioning, Operation, Qualification and Maintenance (PDA, 2010).

12.6.3.9.4.8   The Physical Characteristics of a Sterilization Cycle   It is important to look at the physical parameters of the cycle like temperature, pressure, calibration, and other physical monitoring parameters. Temperature distribution studies and heat penetration studies are conducted using temperature monitoring devices, usually thermocouples. The thermocouples selected for use should be appropriate for the temperature range being monitored. Some companies choose to use resistance temperature detectors (RTDs), because they have a higher level of accuracy than thermocouples. However, thermocouples are less expensive, have a faster response time, and they are made to withstand the "abuse" they get during validation studies. The thermocouples selected for use must be calibrated and accurate to a specified level for the temperature range in which they will be used (Agalloco, 2008; Moldenhauer, 2013 and 2014).

Care should be taken when placing the thermocouples in the sterilizer load for validation. When placing temperature distribution probes, it is important that the probes are not coming into contact with other surfaces that may produce results that are not representative of the temperature in the sterilizer chamber. Placement of heat penetration probes also requires care. The probes should be placed within items in such a way that they do not block off the path of steam penetration to the item. Additionally, the placement of the probes must not create artificial openings where steam could penetrate the item in a way that is not possible in routine sterilization. For thermocouples that have wires which attach to the data recorder, one must also be sure to position the wires so that they do not become damaged by the handling of the load being placed into or out of the sterilizer. The operation of some sterilizers makes it difficult to utilize wired probes as part of the validation process, e.g., probes that operate through a tunnel or probes in sterilizers that rotate or agitate. There are probes that have been designed to wirelessly provide the temperature data to the data logger (Moldenhauer, 2013 and 2014).

Some sterilizers also utilize load probes. These probes are permanently installed in the sterilizer and monitor temperature in both validation and routine production cycles. When installed, the temperature values for these probes are also monitored during the validation cycle (Moldenhauer, 2013 and 2014).

For sterilizers that utilize recirculating water for cooling, thermocouples are also used to assess the temperatures attained in the water prior to initiation of the cooling process. There is an expectation that the water be sterilized during the cycle so that the water used for cooling of the product is sterile (Moldenhauer, 2013 and 2014).

Sterilizer pressure is monitored in moist heat sterilization cycles. The pressure has lesser importance than temperature, but it is used to ensure that saturated steam is used during the exposure dwell period. There are some regulators who routinely check the temperatures observed on recording charts to the expected pressure readings from steam tables. Pressure can play a significant role in ensuring functional product at the completion of the cycle. For example, inadequate overpressure in a plastic cycle may result in deformed containers (Moldenhauer, 2013 and 2014).

The key instrumentation for monitoring or recording temperature and pressure data for the sterilizer should be calibrated in such a way that the calibration can be traced to a recognized national standard. Additionally, the thermocouples used in the validation should be calibrated before and after each study (Moldenhauer, 2013 and 2014).

It is possible to utilize a physical or chemical indicator and/or a physical/chemical integrator to monitor the sterilization cycle. There are a variety of indicators available for different types of sterilization. One of the simplest types of indicators is the use of autoclave tape, which changes color if the tape has been processed in the sterilizer. It does not provide information on the quality of the cycle, and in many cases, does not indicate whether a complete cycle was performed. Physical/chemical integrators assess the process conditions in the cycle, typically integrating the effects of multiple process parameters and provide some guidance on the cycle delivered. One such integrator provides a line showing whether a minimum F_0 value was achieved in the cycle. Neither indicators nor integrators are to be utilized in place of biological indicators. They do provide useful information, like indicating that a load has been processed through the sterilizer (Moldenhauer, 2013 and 2014).

12.6.3.9.4.9   Selecting an Approach for Sterilization Validation   There are established models or approaches that can be used to determine the sterilizer validation criteria like minimum lethality that must be met. In the past, there were three models based upon the thermal death time curve, an overkill model, a combined biological indicator – bioburden based model, and an absolute bioburden model. The key differences in these models are the amount of heat delivered to the product, the effect on stability of the product and the cost of the sterilization cycle (e.g., the utilities used). The Parenteral Drug Association (PDA) reissued their technical report on moist heat sterilization and converted the combined biological indicator-bioburden based model and the absolute bioburden model into a product specific approach to cycle design (PDA, 2007). The intent of each model or approach is to determine the lethality required to deliver the desired probability of a non-sterile unit (Moldenhauer, 2013 and 2014).

The semi-logarithmic survivor curve model can be used to determine the appropriate PNSU, which in most cases is 10^{-6}. This can be expressed as shown in Equation 12.4.

$$Log\,N_F = -F/D + Log\,N_0 \qquad (12.4)$$

In order to determine the lethality that is required for a specific sterilization cycle, this equation can be rearranged to solve for the F-value, as shown in Equation 12.5 (PDA, 2007)

$$F = \left(Log\,N_0 - Log\,N_F\right) \times D_T \qquad (12.5)$$

Where N_0 represents the starting population of the biological challenge organism, e.g., 10^6. The D-value is specific for the microorganism chosen as the biological indicator. N_F represents the final population of microorganisms, which is usually 10^{-6}, or the desired probability of a non-sterile unit (Moldenhauer, 2014).

An overkill cycle provides the most heat to the items being sterilized. It has the highest cost associated with use of the sterilizer. This added heat has an impact on the stability of the item following sterilization. This type of cycle provides a high level of sterility assurance regardless of the level of bioburden present and regardless of the heat resistance of that bioburden. It is assumed that the starting population of bioburden is 10^6, with a $D_{121°C}$ of at least 1 minute, and a z-value of $10°C$. To have a PNSU of 10^{-6}, that would indicate a final biological population or N_F that is 10^{-6}. These values can be entered into the equation to determine the F-value, i.e., the expected lethality. This calculation is shown below using Equation 12.6 (PDA, 2007; Moldenhauer, 2014).

$$F_0 = D_{121°C} \times \left(Log\,N_0 - Log\,N_F\right) \qquad (12.6)$$

$$F_0 = 1.0\,minute - \left(Log\,10^6 - Log\,10^{-6}\right) = 12\,minutes$$

Within the definition of overkill in the PDA's Technical Report (PDA, 2007), an overkill cycle must deliver a lethality of at least 12 minutes under the specified conditions. The PDA's Technical Report (PDA, 2007) added to this definition stating: "a cycle designed with the overkill design approach can be defined as a sterilization cycle that is demonstrated to deliver an $F_{Biological}$ and $F_{Physical}$ of at least 12 minutes to the items being sterilized." (Moldenhauer, 2013 and 2014).

These terms have been defined by PDA to mean (PDA, 2007):

$F_{Physical}$ is defined as the term used to describe the delivered lethality calculated based on the physical parameters of the cycle. The $F_{physical}$-value is calculated as the integration of the lethal rate (L) over time. The lethal rate is calculated per a reference temperature (T_{ref}) and z-value using the equation: $L = 10^{(T-Tref/z)}$. This typically refers to the data obtained from the temperature measurement devices, e.g., heat penetration probes.

$F_{Biological}$ is defined as a term used to describe the delivered lethality measured in terms of actual kill of microbiological organisms on or in a BI challenge system. The

$F_{Biological}$-value is calculated as the $D_T \times LR$, where D_T is the D-value of the BI system at the reference temperature, T, and LR is the actual log reduction of the BI population achieved during the cycle (PDA, 2007).

The change to add the requirements for $F_{Biological}$ to the definition of an overkill cycle was a change over previous definitions. Few companies prior to this time routinely monitored or assessed $F_{Biological}$ as part of their routine qualification requirements. For many companies who had cycles in place for many years, converting to this definition of an overkill cycle necessitated repeating or revising the cycle development studies previously conducted (Moldenhauer, 2013 and 2014).

There is a separate definition of overkill cycles within the European regulations. In the European regulations and compendia for terminally sterilized dosage forms, an overkill cycle is specified as sterilization by moist heat at 121°C for at least 15 minutes (PDA, 2007; Moldenhauer, 2013 and 2014).

It is common to expect that an overkill cycle model be used for the sterilization of equipment and components utilized in aseptic manufacturing operations. It is possible to use this type of sterilization model for some terminal sterilization activities, providing that the items being sterilized can withstand the cycle conditions (Moldenhauer, 2013 and 2014).

Overkill terminal sterilization cycles are too harsh for many products in the pharmaceutical environment. Terminal sterilization is desired for pharmaceutical products as a method to provide for patient safety. Since many overkill cycles are too harsh, alternative models have been developed for those products with some thermal sensitivity, which are called product specific models or approaches. (Older texts refer to these types of approaches as combined biological indicator-bioburden based, or absolute bioburden based cycles.) With this type of approach, one must sufficiently reduce the microbial population to an acceptable level of sterility assurance while maintaining the product's attributes. In order to accomplish this, the models take into account the starting population of the microorganisms' present (bioburden) and the heat resistance of those organisms, along with provision of a safety factor. These values are utilized in the calculation to determine the minimum lethality. Use of this type of model requires the manufacturer to commit to ongoing monitoring of the product bioburden and its heat resistance. An example of the product specific design model calculations is illustrated using Equation 12.6 (PDA, 2007; Moldenhauer, 2013 and 2014).

Manufacturing site data for bioburden indicated:

$$N_0 < 25 \text{ resistant organisms per unit of product}$$

$$D_{121°C} < 0.3 \text{ minutes}$$

In order to add a safety factor, the following values were used:

$$N_0 = 10^2$$

$$D_{121°C} = 0.4 \text{ minutes}$$

The desired PNSU was determined to be 10^{-6}

$$F_{121°C} = \left(\text{Log}\,10^2 - \text{Log}\,10^{-6}\right) \times D_{121°C} = 3.2\,\text{minutes}$$

The above example indicates that the model would deliver the desired PNSU using a F_0 of 3.2 minutes. However, many regulators would expect that additional precautions be established in support of cycles with an F_0 less than 6 minutes, e.g., aseptic filling prior to terminal sterilization or other methods designed to ensure microbiological control (Moldenhauer, 2013 and 2014).

12.6.3.9.4.10 Validating Moist Heat Sterilization Systems The equipment qualification refers to an assessment of the hardware/software used for the sterilization process. It does not address the actual sterilization cycle or the items being processed in the sterilizer. The equipment qualification includes verifying the proper installation of the equipment as well as verifying that it is operating correctly, prior to assessing its capability to sterilize the desired components, equipment or product. These activities are conducted in the installation qualification (IQ), the operational qualification (OQ) or in a combined document that cover the installation and operation qualification (I/OQ). Whether the protocols are combined or separate documents frequently is a function of how complex the equipment qualification process is. The same requirements apply in either case (Moldenhauer, 2013 and 2014).

- *Installation Qualification (IQ)*: In some cases, companies contract with the vendor of the equipment to perform this testing. It is good practice for end-user personnel participate in this activity, even when the vendor conducts the studies to gain knowledge of the system. The documentation generated becomes a technical handbook for the system as supplied to your site. This information can be invaluable when determining at a later date whether replacement parts are or are not identical to those installed. It is at the end-user's discretion on whether the hardware and software are tested concurrently or as separate documents (Moldenhauer, 2003). Some other considerations include (Moldenhauer, 2013 and 2014); verification that items match the purchase order, no damage in shipping, all items received, supporting documentation received, and so forth.

  It is beneficial to make this document as comprehensive and detailed as possible. This document becomes the technical handbook for the sterilizer over time. It is especially useful when trying to assess the appropriateness of replacement parts, and whether they are equivalent to the original installation (Moldenhauer, 2013 and 2014).
- *Operational Qualification (OQ):* allows you to assess whether the system it operates at the specified conditions, prior to adding the influence of the item to be sterilized into the mix. It may also be called the dynamic equipment qualification. Once you initiate sterilization of items within the unit, if a problem occurs it is not clear whether it is the sterilizer performance

at fault or effects of the item in the sterilizer. The OQ of the hardware and the software or control system may be performed within a single document or in separate documents. The utilities used to support the sterilization system, e.g., clean steam, oil-free compressed air, and the like should be qualified either concurrent with the OQ or prior to the OQ being conducted (Moldenhauer, 2013 and 2014).

- *Empty Chamber Temperature Distribution:* Studies are conducted using temperature distribution probes, usually arranged in a fixed or geometric pattern, to evaluate the uniformity of heat delivered within the sterilizer chamber. For this study type, fixed patterns are used most often. This allows for direct comparison of data from one study to another, which is useful when these studies are used following production deficiencies. Unless heat is delivered to all areas of the sterilizer chamber, one cannot ensure that all of the items in the sterilizer will be appropriately sterilized in the cycle. During these studies it is common to find that some of the sterilizer parameters may need to be modified, for example the bleeder valves, water spray nozzle directions, directional air flow, and so forth. The data obtained from these studies is also used as baseline data for evaluating the sterilizer's performance characteristics over the life of the sterilizer. Penetration probes are not typically used in these evaluations. It is important that the temperature distribution probes are properly located and that they do not come into contact with either the sterilizer trays or the sterilizer itself (Moldenhauer, 2013 and 2014).

- *Software Evaluations:* During the OQ, it is also common to evaluate several features of the control system including for example: Verification that it sequences properly through the various stages of the sterilization cycle, alarms trigger as designed, security features are enabled, all documentation required in the URS is present, stored records are retrievable, records are accurate, and so forth (Moldenhauer, 2014).

- *Sterilization Cycle Development:* After the OQ, is complete, verifying that the sterilizer is operating correctly, cycle development studies are initiated. The requirements may differ somewhat for sterilization of porous/hard good loads and those for terminal sterilization of liquids, or for dry heat sterilization in ovens or tunnels. The PDA's Technical Report Number 1 (PDA, 2007) provides a decision tree that walks through the various evaluations that should be considered in assessing the process type to be used for moist heat sterilization. This document also indicates which parameters should be established for each different process type of cycle (Moldenhauer, 2013 and 2014).

Cycle development studies should be used to determine the physical parameters required to appropriately sterilize the component, equipment or final product. This includes placing the item into a specified loading pattern, except for dry heat tunnels. Part of this process is to determine a range of acceptable parameters that may be met in performing the studies. The result of this process should be an item that is sterile and functional post sterilization. Studies for cycle development should be formally documented (PDA, 2007; Moldenhauer, 2014).

- *Pre-Qualification Activities:* To conduct cycle development studies, it is important to conduct some evaluations prior to the actual cycle development like determination of slowest-to-heat location and slowest-to-heat zone (of a liquid).

Determination of the slowest-to-heat location is important. When performing validation studies using the selected items is where to place the penetration probes to measure the item's temperature accurately. Additionally, one wants to monitor at the "cold spot" of the item, to ensure that the entire item has seen the recorded temperature (at minimum). As such, it is necessary to perform studies that assess the heating characteristics of the item. These studies may also be called component-mapping studies. Many components, especially within equipment loads, are complex and it would take numerous probes to determine all of the "cold spots". To minimize the number of probes and studies required, some assessment is conducted to evaluate those spots expected to be more difficult to heat, like those with the greatest mass, potential for entrapped air, long hoses, and those items that encompass combinations of these types of concerns. There are differences in evaluating "cold spots" for those items which present issues in removing air versus those that have a high mass. If air removal is the concern, then the probes would be placed within the wrapped item so that the tip of the probe is adjacent to the item, so that one can determine the equilibration time. The equilibration time represents the effectiveness of the air removal. Items with a significant mass tend to have a temperature lag to the sterilizer chamber temperature, due to the energy transfer not the temperature in the sterilizer chamber. As such, the probes should be placed to measure the heat penetration in contact with the item. This information aids in the determination of the load come-up time. It is not required to do these studies in each sterilizer, or even in a production sterilizer. It just should use the same type of sterilization process (PDA, 2007; Moldenhauer, 2013 and 2014).

Mapping studies are also performed for liquid-filled containers. It is assumed that these studies are not required for containers of 50 mL size or smaller, due to the small size of the container. The studies usually look at different levels of solution within the container as illustrated in Figure 12.5 (Moldenhauer, 2014).

D-value studies should be conducted. They are affected by: the size of the inoculum, type of organism, sporulation and growth media composition, pH, phase of spore maturity, and incubation temperature for recovery of organisms. The surface on which the biological indicator is placed can have an affect the heat resistance of the biological indicator. For example, placing a biological indicator on the surface of a porous rubber stopper, can have increased heat resistance, since the biological indicator is protected by the porosity of the stopper and the poor transfer of heat from the rubber. In general, we assume that placement on a glass or stainless steel surface does not affect the D-value sufficiently to be of concern. Biological indicators placed on paper carriers, can show different resistance based upon the quality of the paper used as a carrier. For porous/hard good loads, one must evaluate the biological indicator's heat resistance when directly inoculated on the rubber stoppers being sterilized. Rubber inherently is a poor conductor of heat. Data has been published to show that the heat resistance is affected by the rubber composition. This effect varies

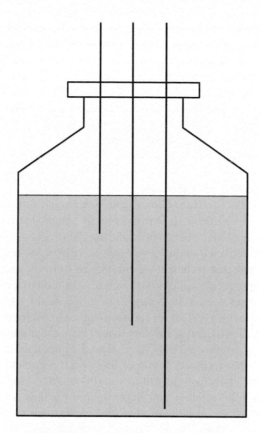

FIGURE 12.5   Example of Mapping in a Liquid Filled Vial.

based upon the specific biological indicator used, the formulation of the stopper, and the types of treatments to which the stopper is subjected (Rubio and Moldenhauer, 1995) As knowledge in this area has increased, concerns have arisen with other items that may change the biological indicator resistance. This has led to companies starting to evaluate the heat resistance of tubing and other materials processed in the load (Moldenhauer, 2013 and 2014).

For liquid loads, the biological indicator should be placed in direct contact with the liquid to determine the D-value. The D-value can change based upon the strain of biological indicator used as well as the formulation of the liquid product. If a carrier is used for the biological indicator, the sterilization cycle design should take into account the D-value on the carrier as well as the D-value determined when in direct contact with the liquid or component being evaluated (Moldenhauer, 2013 and 2014).

- *Determination of the Selected Loading Configuration (Load Patterns):* Typical considerations include: the necessary capacity required to support production activities as well as ensure that effectiveness of the sterilization process can be achieved. For example, if a water spray cycle is used, the loading should allow for adequate drainage of the water that contacts the items being sterilized. When sterilizing hard goods, many of the items need to be wrapped in sterilization wrap to protect the sterile surfaces until they are used. If sterilization wrap is used, it should be non-shedding, and provide a microbial barrier (keeping the item sterile). The amount of wrapping should not be excessive, as this can reduce the effectiveness of air removal, steam penetration, and temperature penetration. Larger mass items should be placed on the lower level of sterilizer trucks, in order to reduce the risk of wetting by condensate. Care should be taken to ensure that condensate from items minimizes drip onto other items. The configurations should be photographed or drawn to be able to reproduce the loading parameters (PDA, 2007; Moldenhauer, 2013 and 2014).

- *Sterilization of Porous/Hard Goods:* Sterilization of porous items in a sterilizer load can be difficult. It is important to ensure that the air normally present in the load items is removed during the process to ensure that the desired heat is delivered to the items being sterilizer. As such, the data generated must show that sufficient air is removed from the chamber and load prior to the exposure conditions of the cycle. Additionally, the air and non-condensable gases need to be removed from the steam supply provided to the sterilizer. It is also critical for saturated steam (must have an appropriate dryness level) be provided to the sterilizer. The number and type of studies required during this process may vary, depending upon the site's knowledge of the items to be sterilized. Some of the typical parameters evaluated as part of this process include the following: (PDA, 2007; Moldenhauer, 2013) Jacket temperature, number and depth of pre-vacuum conditions, steam pulse levels, time and conditions for chamber heat-up, exposure time and temperature, allowable time for cooling (exhaust phase) and drying, and air breaks. It is useful to standardize cycles to aid in reducing the ongoing validation and revalidation costs (Moldenhauer, 2014).

- *Sterilization of Liquid Loads:* In a liquid load, the liquid inside of the container is heated by the transfer of heat from the outside of the container. The water contents steam and provide the sterilant inside the container. Non-aqueous solutions, like suspensions and emulsions, require use of a rotation or agitation cycle to keep the load in motion. Several types of sterilization processes may be used including saturated steam, overpressure cycles, steam-air mixtures, and superheated water. For many liquid cycles air removal is not performed, however it is important to ensure that a system is used to ensure uniform heat distribution within the chamber. The containers in a load heat do not necessarily heat at the same rate. Items closer to the outside may heat more quickly than items in the center of the load. The concern is to be sure that the items receiving the least heat are sterile and the items which receive the most heat are not adversely affected from a functional and stability point of view (PDA, 2007; Moldenhauer, 2013 and 2014).

- *Determining the Cycle Parameters to Use:* The parameters to measure in a sterilization cycle are dependent upon the type of items to be sterilized, e.g., porous/hard goods loads, terminal sterilization loads, dry heat sterilization, or dry heat depyrogenation. In addition, one must also determine the criticality of these parameters. Some parameters are so important, frequently deemed critical parameters that when they are not met the sterilization cycle should be deemed unacceptable. Other parameters, while important may be mitigated, for example a pressure failure at some parts of the cycle might be mitigated by 100% inspection of the load for a type of physical defect. The PDA's Technical Report Number 1, provides a listing of process parameters to be considered for moist heat sterilization of porous loads including (PDA, 2007): Jacket temperature and/or pressure, number and depth of vacuum pulses prior to exposure, level of the steam charge, number and requirements for positive pressure pulses, chamber come-up time, exposure time, exposure temperature set-point, temperature of the chamber drain during exposure, chamber temperature during exposure, allowable temperature range for the load probe during exposure, chamber pressure during exposure, minimum allowable F_0 during exposure, allowable time for the load to cool down after exposure, drying time after exposure, and the rate for vacuum breaks. Depending upon the sterilizer configuration used, not all of the stated parameters are applicable (Moldenhauer, 2013 and 2014).

The PDA's Technical Report Number 1, provides a listing of process parameters to be considered for liquid-filled moist heat sterilization loads including: (PDA, 2007) jacket temperature and/or pressure, fan rotations per minute during the cycle, agitation rate during the cycle, water flow rate during the cycle, chamber water level prior to exposure, heat-up time prior to exposure, temperature heat-up rate prior to exposure, rate of temperature heat-up prior to exposure, pressure ramp-up rate prior to exposure, temperature set-point during exposure, exposure time, chamber pressure during exposure, redundant heating media temperature during exposure, load probe temperature(s) during exposure, minimum allowable F_0 for the load probe during exposure, minimum allowable F_0 for the load probe post exposure, temperature cool-down rate post exposure, pressure ramp-down rate post exposure, load cool-down rate, and maximum allowable load probe accumulated F_0 post exposure. Note: while PDA expresses this term post exposure, some companies actually calculate the value accumulated only in the exposure period. The applicability of these parameters is determined by the type of sterilization process selected (Moldenhauer, 2013 and 2014).

- *Performance Qualification (PQ):* The purpose of the performance qualification (PQ) studies is to demonstrate that the sterilization process consistently meets its pre-defined requirements. A minimum of three acceptable studies is required. If minimum and maximum loads are performed, a minimum of three studies of for each load configuration are performed. There are some provisions for bracketing of load configurations, e.g., qualification of the maximum and minimum container size may justify the elimination of testing for intermediate container sizes. The IQ and OQ should be successfully completed prior to initiating the PQ studies. Supporting systems like utilities necessary for the process should also have been completed by this time (Moldenhauer, 2013 and 2014).

The PQ includes both physical and biological qualification of the sterilizer load. It is common practice to perform the studies concurrently. For moist heat sterilization, the physical qualification data yields an $F_{Physical}$-value while the biological data yields a $F_{Biological}$-value. These values should be correlated to ensure that both the physical and biological parameters for the cycle design have been met. The studies should be performed at "worst case" conditions (Moldenhauer, 2013 and 2014).

12.6.3.9.4.11   Challenges for Porous Load Cycles   Traditionally *Geobacillus stearothermophilus* is used as the challenge organism in this type of cycle. The typical cycle design utilizes an overkill approach. Data should be generated using the biological indicators directly inoculated onto the items or carriers may be used. Carriers are available in a variety of formats including: paper, wire, stainless steel, aluminum or other appropriate materials. The biological indicators should be placed in the most difficult to sterilize areas of the item. Some examples include: within long tubing, areas where it is difficult to achieve air removal and/or steam penetration, within the pleats of filter cartridges, and so forth. When these studies are performed concurrently with physical qualification, care must be taken to ensure that placement of thermocouples does not impact either the air removal or the steam penetration such that the biological challenge is seeing different conditions than if the probes were not in position. Biological challenge studies should be performed for both minimum and maximum load configurations (PDA, 2007; Moldenhauer, 2013 and 2014).

12.6.3.9.4.12   Sterilizer Equivalence   Equivalence can be addressed with different types of evaluations. One consideration is the ability to use sterilization data from one sterilizer in the qualification of another sterilizer. While this has been accepted by some regulatory bodies, there is an expectation that the sterilizers use the same sterilization process, have the same physical size, construction and basic operation. It is expected, these sterilizers should be in the same general location, e.g., the same plant although maybe not in direct proximity of each other. In this scenario, each sterilizer would be tested to ensure that the operation of the sterilizer is within the expected norms prior to utilizing data from another sterilizer for qualification (Agalloco, 2008; Moldenhauer, 2013 and 2014).

12.6.3.9.4.13   Equivalence of Different Containers/Fill Volumes   Evaluating minor differences in container dimensions and/or in the fill volumes within a container can be accomplished by performing side-by-side statistical evaluation of the heat penetration in both containers (or fill volumes). A test like a Student T-test may be used for this evaluation (Moldenhauer, 2013 and 2014).

12.6.3.9.4.14   Equivalence of Different Load Configurations   When evaluating changes to the load configurations for moist heat sterilization porous loads or hard good loads, the heat penetration data can be compared between the two load configurations in both the minimum and maximum loading arrangement. This evaluation may include a statistical evaluation of the data also (Moldenhauer, 2013 and 2014).

12.6.4 DRY HEAT STERILIZATION

Sterilization cycles utilize hot, dry air to accomplish sterilization. These processes have not been extensively. Different opinions exist regarding the predictive nature of the microbial destruction or endotoxin reduction in dry heat cycles. Some choose to perform calculations to assess the lethality delivered and the theoretical endotoxin reduction while others challenge these calculations. The calculations used to determine the theoretical reduction of endotoxin are limited by the various D- and z-values used in the calculation. Since there is not a single acceptable D and z-value, the calculations yield a variety of results depending upon the value utilized (Agalloco, 2008; Moldenhauer, 2013 and 2014).

Since one log of endotoxin reduction requires substantially more heat than what is required for inactivation of biological indicators, biological indicators are not typically required as the endotoxin reduction provides more challenge to the system that the destruction of the biological indicator (PDA Technical Report Number 1, 2007). For those studies which must show depyrogenation in addition to sterilization, the endotoxin challenge should show a minimum three-log reduction of endotoxin (Moldenhauer, 2013 and 2014).

Dry heat sterilizers are available in both batch and continuous configurations. Continuous configurations typically have a tunnel (Moldenhauer, 2014).

12.6.4.1 Dry Heat Ovens

Validation is conducted in a similar fashion to moist heat sterilizers. Studies are performed measuring temperature distribution, heat penetration, and biological (or endotoxin) challenges. The F_0 calculation for moist heat is not appropriate when using dry heat. For depyrogenation, in place of this calculation the F_H calculation (some groups call this F_P) is used. It uses the same type of F_0 calculation, but the reference temperature is set at 250°C and the z-value is set at 46.4°C (PDA TR 3 [revised], 2013c) (Note: some authors prefer the use of a z-value of 47.6°C from the Tsuji and Lewis article.) If sterilization is the only objective of the cycle, spores of *Bacillus atrophaeus* are typically used as biological indicators in the cycle (Moldenhauer, 2014).

If the oven is used for sterilization only, the F_H calculation utilizes a reference temperature of 160°C and a z-value of 20°C (PDA TR3 [revised], 2013c).

12.6.4.2 Worst Case Conditions

The oven validation studies are conducted using worst case conditions. Typically, this is accomplished by reducing the exposure time and/or temperature (Moldenhauer, 2014).

12.6.4.3 Load Size and Configuration

Dry heat sterilization is not as effective as moist heat sterilization since the hot air may not be able to account for differences in the loading. The loading configurations should be established and tightly controlled. It has been documented that in some cases minimum loads received lesser amounts of heat delivered than in the corresponding maximum load (Agalloco, 2008). The condensation of saturated steam delivers a greater amount of heat to the product than is available in a dry heat oven. Based upon some of the reported variations, every load configuration should be validated. Some companies still try to use minimum and maximum loading (Moldenhauer, 2013 and 2014).

12.6.4.4 Monitoring of Cycles

Typical parameters monitored for dry heat sterilization cycles include: exposure time and temperature, cooling time or final temperature, information on the blowers used, and so forth (Moldenhauer, 2013).

12.6.4.5 Dry Heat Depyrogenation (and Sterilization) Tunnels

Tunnels allow for continuous dry heat sterilization, with the item traveling on a belt through the sterilization process. They are validated in much the same way as a dry heat oven. Key validation parameters are the belt speed (which corresponds to the amount of time the item is subjected to the sterilization process) and the exposure set-point temperature. Biological indicators are not routinely used in these cycles, since the intent is to perform depyrogenation. The endotoxin challenge units should be prepared directly inoculating the endotoxin onto the surface of the items to be processed in the tunnel. Data should be available to show the level of the challenge is sufficient to assess a minimum three-log reduction of endotoxin. Additionally, it is important to develop data on the recovery efficiency for the endotoxin method. For example, it might look like a total reduction of endotoxin occurred, when in reality the method was not appropriate to show the recovery of endotoxin from the surface of the item (Moldenhauer, 2013 and 2014).

12.6.4.6 Loading

Dry heat sterilization using a continuous process does not have the same type of loading configuration or arrangement as is possible with a batch sterilizer. The items are "pushed" into the sterilizer process on the conveyor belt. In most cases, those units at the beginning and trailing edges of the items typically represent the worst case conditions (Agalloco, 2008; Moldenhauer, 2013 and 2014).

It is common for many companies to bracket the loading qualification with the largest and smallest size item sterilized. Intermediate sizes are not routinely challenged. However, the company should have a plan ready to explain why the intermediate sizes do not require qualification.

12.6.4.7 Worst Case Challenges

During validation a company may lower the conveyor belt speed (exposure time) and/or the exposure temperature. Some companies qualify at nominal temperatures. When this occurs, they do not have the necessary data to show effective sterilization at the minimum allowable conditions unless nominal production is routinely performed at the minimum conditions (Moldenhauer, 2014).

12.6.4.8   Validating Dry Heat Sterilization Processes

There are both similarities and differences to other sterilization processes for validation.

- *Equipment Qualification:* The PDA's Technical Report Number 3 (revised) (2013) provides detailed instructions for equipment qualification. Some of the considerations at this stage include: electrical program logic, verification of alarms, item interlocks overload, door interlocks, gasket integrity, air balance, vibration analysis, louver balance ability, louver position, gate balance ability, blower rotation, blower revolutions per minute (RPM), heater elements, room balance, temperature sensors, and belt speed. Other concerns include environmental qualification, uniformity of heating media, and empty chamber temperature distribution studies (Moldenhauer, 2014).
- *Process Development:* Overkill approaches are typically used for sterilization. The probability of a non-sterile unit is calculated using the following calculation: (PDA TR 3 [revised], 2013 and Moldenhauer, 2014)

$$\text{Log PNSU} = -F_H / D + \text{Log} N_0$$

where:

F_H = lowest F_H in the load
D = $D_{160°C}$ value of the biological indicator
N_0 = Initial population of the biological indicator

If the $F_H = 60$ minutes, the initial population is 10^6 and the D-value at 160°C is two minutes, the calculation would be as follows:

$$\text{Log PNSU} = -60 / 2 + 6$$

$$\text{Log PNSU} = -30 + 6$$

$$\text{Log PNSU} = -24$$

$$\text{PNSU} = 10^{-24}$$

There are allowances for a product-specific design approach, and a minimum PNSU of 10^{-6} (PDA TR 3 [revised] 2013).

During this phase of the project, the operating parameters are defined and typically include: time and temperature during heat-up and cooling, pressure differentials, temperature during exposure, and exposure time (belt speed for tunnel systems). It should also include a specified PNSU. Studies should be performed to confirm the assumptions made (PDA TR 3 [revised] 2013 and Moldenhauer, 2014).

For batch processes, loading patterns should be determined and based upon data obtained in temperature distribution and heat penetration studies. Typically, the both types of probe and the BI or endotoxin challenge are placed adjacent to each other. Consideration in these studies include: maximum variation in distribution probe measurements (probe to probe and within a probe), maximum difference in temperature between the probes and the controller set-point, and minimum F_H (PDA TR3 [revised] 2013 and Moldenhauer, 2014).

For tunnels, the worst case load for each temperature should be determined, typically by calculating throughput of items (mass/time), belt speed/item passage time, and the weight of the items in the load (capacity). After determining the worst case parameters, the most mass container per unit area is selected, the belt speed is set to the maximum for any container and the tunnel is loaded at the maximum rate (PDA TR3 [revised] 2013; Moldenhauer, 2014).

- *Performance Qualification Studies:* These studies should include physical qualification and biological qualification of the load (either biological indicators or endotoxin units) (PDA TR3 [revised] 2013 and Moldenhauer, 2014).
- Provisions are provided for process equivalency based upon the chamber or tunnel size and configuration, airflow dynamics, temperature come-up and uniformity, conveyor speed, temperature equilibration time, and materials of construction. Other concerns are load configurations, temperature distribution, F_H values, biological inactivation, and the heat-up and cool-down rates (PDA TR3 [revised] 2013; Moldenhauer, 2014).

12.7   SYSTEMS TO MAINTAIN STERILIZER QUALIFICATION

12.7.1   PERSONNEL TRAINING

Sterilizers are expensive and complex pieces of equipment. It is important that the individuals operating this equipment be thoroughly trained. Some companies have established certification programs for sterilizer operators.

Documentation requirements to be included in the training are: e.g., SOPs, Protocols. All of the activities surrounding the validation of sterilizers should be thoroughly documented. This may be in the form of protocols or standard operating procedures (SOPs) that govern the process (Moldenhauer, 2014).

12.7.1.1   Summary Report

Final reports should be generated and approved at the completion of each phase of the validation testing. This report should be accurate, complete, and approved by those organizations that approved the protocol (Moldenhauer, 2014).

12.7.1.2   Ongoing Activities

Once validated, it is important to maintain the sterilizer within its qualified parameters. As such, it is important to monitor the sterilizer's performance. Some of the evaluations should include review of the cycle parameters during routine use, evaluation of deviations that occur, review of maintenance activities, and change control. Should a significant number of deviations occur, one must consider whether there are additional parameters that should be added for evaluation in routine qualification to better control the sterilizer's performance. Requalification should be conducted on a periodic basis, as well as when deemed necessary by maintenance or other activities (Moldenhauer, 2013 and 2014).

12.8 CONCLUSION

Sterilization in any of the various forms described provide an important method to aid in the contamination control of a process. Within the types of sterilization, terminal sterilization of the product in its final closed container provides the highest level of control and prevention of contamination.

REFERENCES

Agalloco, J. (1993) The validation life cycle. *Journal of Parenteral Science and Technology.* **47**(3): 142–147.

Agalloco, J. (2008) Sterilization Process Validation. In *Microbiology in Pharmaceutical Manufacturing.* Second Edition, Volume 1. Richard Prince, Ed. PDA/DHI. Bethesda, MD. 401–423.

ANSI (2012) ANSI/AAMI/ISO 13408-5: 2006/(R)2012. Aseptic Processing of Health Care Products – Part 5: Sterilization in Place. American National Standard.

ANSI (2009) ANSI/AAMI/ISO TIR 17665-2: 2009. Sterilization of Health Care Products – Moist Heat – Part 2: Guidance on the Application of ANSI/AAMI/ISO 17665-1. American National Standard.

Bharati, S., et al. (2009). Studies on a Novel Bioactive Glass and Composite Coating with Hydroxyapatite on Titanium Based Alloys: Effect of Y-Sterilization on Coating. *Journal of the European Ceramic Society* 29(12): 2527–35.

Bryce, D. M. (1956) Tests for the Sterility of Pharmaceutical Preparations; the Design and Interpretation of Sterility Tests. Journal of Pharmacy and Pharmacology: 561-572.

DeSantis, P. (2008) Steam Sterilization in Autoclaves. In *Validation of Pharmaceutical Processes Third Edition.* Agalloco, J. and Carleton, F. J., Eds. Informa Healthcare USA, Inc. New York. 175–186.

European Committee for Standardization (2009) *BS EN 285:2006 + A2:2009 Sterilization – Steam Sterilizers – Large Sterilizers.* Brussels.

European Union (2001) Final Version of Annex 15 to the EU Guide to Good Manufacturing Practice. Working Party on Control of Medicines and Inspections. Brussels. Downloaded from www.it-asso.com/gxp/eudralex_v21/contents/vol-4/pdfs-en/v4an 15.pdf on July 15, 2011.

European Agency for the Evaluation of Medicinal Products (EMEA) (2000) *Decision Trees for the Selection of Sterilisation Methods* (CPMP/QWP/054/98). EMEA Evaluation of Medicines for Human Use. Committee for Proprietary Medicinal Products (CPMP), London.

European Commission (2008 revised) EU Guidelines to Good Manufacturing Practice Medicinal Products for Human and Veterinary Products Annex 1 (Corrected). EudraLex The Rules Governing Medicinal Products in the European Union. Volume 4. (Implementation by March 2010). Brussels, Belgium.

Eylath, Amnon, et al. (2003) Successful Sterilization Using Chlorine Dioxide Gas part One: Sanitizing an Aseptic Fill Isolator. *BioProcess International.* Downloaded from: file: ///C:/DocLib/Literature/Chlorine%20Dioxide/Morrisey%20-%20Aseptic%20Isolato r.pdf on January 4, 2018.

FDA (1994a) *Guidelines on the Principles of Process Validation.* March. Rockville, MD.

FDA (1994b) *Guidance for Industry for the Submission Documentation for Sterilization Process Validation in Applications for Human and Veterinary Drug Products.* Rockville, MD.

FDA (1997) Hazard Analysis and Critical Control Point Principles and Application Guidelines (HACCP). National Advisory Committee on Microbiological Criteria for Foods. Downloaded from www.cfsan.fda.gov/~comm/nacmcfp.html

FDA (2003) 21CFR§211.113b. Control of Microbiological Contamination. GMP Publications, Inc.

FDA (2004) Guidance for Industry: Sterile Drug Products Produced by Aseptic Processing – Current Good Manufacturing Practice. U.S. Health and Human Services. Food and Drug Association. (CBER) Office of Regulatory Affairs (ORA). Pharmaceutical CGMPs.

Food and Drug Administration (FDA) (1976) *Proposed Current Good Manufacturing Practices for Large Volume Parenterals (LVP GMPs).* Drafted 1976 and subsequently withdrawn 1993. Rockville, MD.

HTM-2010 (1994) *Part 3: Validation and Verification.* Her Majesty's Stationary Office.

International Organization for Standardization (ISO) (2006) ISO 17665-1:2006 Sterilization of Health Care Products – Moist Heat – Part 1. Requirements for the Development, Validation and Routine Control of a Sterilization Process for Medical Devices. Geneva, Switzerland.

ISO (2007) ISO 11135:2007 Sterilization of Health Care Products—Ethylene Oxide—Part 1: Requirements for Development, Validation, and Routine Control of a Sterilization Process for Medical Devices. Geneva, Switzerland.

ISO (2008) ISO 10993-7 Biological evaluation of medical devices, part 7: ethylene oxide sterilization residuals. International Organisation for Standardisation. Geneva, Switzerland.

ISO (2012) ANSI/AAMI/ISO 13408-2006(r)2012 Aseptic Processing of Health Care Products – Part 5: Sterilization in Place. Geneva, Switzerland.

ISO (2013) ISO 17665-3:2013 Sterilization of Health Care Products – Moist Heat – Part 3: Guidance on the Designation of a Medical Device to a Product Family and Processing Category for Steam Sterilization. Geneva, Switzerland.

Knudsen, L. F. (1949) Sample Size of Parenteral Solutions for Sterility Testing. *Journal of the American Pharmacists Association* 38: 332–337

Lowe, J., et al. (2013) Impact of Chlorine Dioxide Gas Sterilization on Nosocomial Organisms Viability in a Hospital Room. *International Journal of Environmental Research and Public Health* 10(6): 2596–2605.

Miller, M. J., et al. (2008) Microbiological Control Strategies During the Development of Pharmaceutical Processes. In *Microbiology in Pharmaceutical Manufacturing* Volume 1. Prince, R., Ed. PDA/DHI Publishers, Bethesda, MD. 237–282.

Moldenhauer, J. (1999) Contributing factors to variability in biological indicator performance data. *PDA Journal of Pharmaceutical Science and Technology* 53(4): 157–162.

Moldenhauer, J. (2011) Personal Communication of Data for *B. smithii.*

Moldenhauer, J. (2013) Validation of Moist and Dry Heat Sterilization. In *Sterile Product Development: Formulation, Process, Quality and Regulatory Considerations. AAPS Advances in the Pharmaceutical Sciences Series 6.* Kolhe, P., Shah, M., and Rathore, N. American Association of Pharmaceutical Sciences and Springer. New York, Heidelberg, Cordrecht, and London. 535–574.

Moldenhauer, J. (2014) Sterilization Processes. In *Contamination Control Volume 2*, Madsen, R. and Moldenhauer, J., Eds. PDA/DHI Publishers. Bethesda, MD.

Oliver, J.D., et al. (1995) Entry into, and Resuscitation from, the Viable but Nonculturable State by *Vibrio Vulnificus* in an Estuarine Environment. *Applied and Environmental Microbiology* (July) 61(7): 2624–2630.

PDA (1981) PDA Technical Report 7 (TR7) Depyrogenation. Bethesda, MD.

PDA (2007) PDA Technical Report 1, Revised 2007, (TR 1) Validation of Moist Heat Sterilization Processes Cycle Design, Development, Qualification and Ongoing Control. Parenteral Drug Association. Bethesda, MD.

PDA (2010) Technical Report No. 48 Moist Heat Sterilizer Systems: Design, Commissioning, Operation, Qualification and Maintenance. Parenteral Drug Association. Bethesda, MD.

PDA (2010) Technical Report No. 48 Moist Heat Sterilizer Systems: Design, Commissioning, Operation, Qualification and Maintenance. Parenteral Drug Association. Bethesda, MD.

PDA (2013a) *Technical Report No. 61 Steam in Place*. Parenteral Drug Association. Bethesda, MD.

PDA (2013b) *Technical Report No.3 (revised 2013) Validation of Dry Heat Processes Used for Depyrogenation and Sterilization*. Parenteral Drug Association. Bethesda, MD.

Pharmaceutical Inspection Convention (PIC/s) (2011) Recommendation on the Validation of Aseptic Processes. PI 007-06.

Pharmaceutical Validation (2011) Biological Process Validation of Dry-Heat Sterilization Cycles. In *Pharmaceutical Validation* Downloaded from http://pharmaceuticalvalidatio n.blogspot.com/2010/01/biological-process-validation-of-dry.html on September 11, 2011.

Rapid Micro Methods (2011) Validating Rapid Micro Methods. Downloaded from http://rap idmicromethods.com/files/validation.html on September 8, 2011.

Rubio, S. L. and Moldenhauer, J. (1995) Effect of Rubber Stopper Composition, Preservative Pretreatment and Rinse Water Temperature on the Moist Heat Resistance of *Bacillus stearothermophilus* ATCC 12980. *PDA Journal of Pharmaceutical Science and Technology* 49(1): 29–31.

Sadowski, M. (2009) The Use of Biological Indicators in the Development and Qualification of Moist Heat Sterilization Processes. In *Biological Indicators for Sterilization Processes*. Gomez, M. and Moldenhauer, J., Eds. PDA/DHI Publishers, Bethesda, MD. 219–270.

Setlow, P. (2009) Bacterial Endospores: Mechanisms that Contribute to their Longevity and Resistance. In *Biological Indicators for Sterilization Processes*. Gomez, M. and Moldenhauer, J., Eds. PDA/DHI Publishers, Bethesda, MD. 25–54.

Stamatis, D. H. (2003) *Failure Mode and Effect Analysis, FMEA from Theory to Execution*, Second Edition. ASQ Quality Press, Milwaukee, WI.

Sutton, S. V. W. and Moldenhauer, J. (2004) Towards an Improved Sterility Test. *PDA Journal of Pharmaceutical Science and Technology* 58(6): 284–286.

United States Pharmacopeia (USP) (2012a) <1229> Sterilization of Compendial Articles, *United States Pharmacopeia, USP 36-NF3*, First Supplement. Pharmacopeial Convention. Rockville, MD.

USP (2012b) <1229.2> Moist Heat Sterilization of Aqueous Liquids. *United States Pharmacopeia, USP 36-NF3*, First Supplement. Pharmacopeial Convention. Rockville, MD.

USP (2013a) <1129.4> Sterilizing Filtration of Liquids. Pharmacopeial Forum (PF Online) 39(2) In Process Revision. New USP37-NF32 1 S. Downloaded from www.usppf.com/ pf/pub/index.html on August 8, 2013.

USP (2013b) <1229.6> Liquid Phase Sterilization. Pharmacopeial Forum (PF Online) 39(4) In Process Revision. New USP 37-NF32 2 S. Downloaded from www.usppf.com/pf/ pub/index.html on August 8, 2013.

USP (2013c) <1229.7> Gaseous Sterilization. Pharmacopeial Forum (PF Online) 39(3). Downloaded from www.usppf.com/pf/pub/index.html on August 8, 2013.

USP (2013d) <1229.8> Dry Heat Sterilization. Pharmacopeial Forum (PF Online) 39(3). Downloaded from www.usppf.com/pf/pub/index.html on August 8, 2013.

USP (2013e) <1229.10 > Radiation Sterilization. Pharmacopeial Forum (PF Online) 39(2). Downloaded from www.usppf.com/pf/pub/index.html on August 8, 2013.USP (2017) <1229.1> Steam Sterilization by Direct Contact. *The United States Pharmacopeial Convention*. Rockville, MD.

Wikipedia (2013) Sterilization (Microbiology). Downloaded from http://en.wikipedia.org/wiki/Sterilization_%28microbiology%29 on August 19, 2013.

Wikipedia (2018) Chlorine Dioxide. Downloaded from: www.bing.com/search?q=chlorine+dioxide+sterilization&qs=n&form=QBLH&sp=-1&pq=chlorine+dioxide+sterilizationš=4-30&sk=&cvid=A72B2982C1FC4508A57DC534BF1F6B4A on January 4, 2018).

Index